When Winter Came

A Country Doctor's Journey to Fight the Flu Pandemic of 1918

MARY BETH SARTOR OBERMEYER

MAYO CLINIC PRESS

MAYO CLINIC PRESS
200 First St. SW
Rochester, MN 55905
MCPress.MayoClinic.org

For bulk sales to employers, member groups and
health-related companies, contact Mayo Clinic at
SpecialSalesMayoBooks@mayo.edu.

ISBN 978-1-945564-15-4

Library of Congress Control Number: 2022942436

Printed in the United States of America

**Proceeds from the sale of Mayo Clinic Press books benefit
medical education and research at Mayo Clinic.**

*This book is published with generous support from
John T. and Lillian G. Mathews,
Founding Benefactors of
Mayo Clinic Heritage Hall*

Welcome

"I am needed." Here is the summary of Dr. Pierre Sartor's life and practice as a prairie physician.

When Winter Came is a fascinating firsthand story of the great influenza pandemic of 1918-1919. It is within the fullness of Dr. Sartor's simple statement that we learn what motivated and steadied him and propelled him to accomplish what he did. His stories invite comparisons and reveal commonalities with our own stories of another pandemic 100 years later — which has taken far more lives, despite medical advances that Dr. Sartor and his contemporaries could never have imagined.

I have been privileged to practice medicine at Mayo Clinic since 1988 and founded the Mayo Vaccine Research Group soon after I arrived. I have devoted my adult life to combatting and preventing infectious diseases with the use of vaccines. For this reason, I identify deeply with the descriptions and struggles of Dr. Sartor in Iowa and Dr. Edward C. Rosenow of the Mayo staff as related in the pages of this book.

Plagues and pandemics have purposes, even though we might not grasp them fully. For Dr. Sartor, and many physicians like him, the virtues of placing others before self, service to one's community, a deep spiritual faith and the determination to serve the needs of the patient were paramount. Indeed, the primary value of Mayo Clinic is as simple as it is profound

4

and was anticipated and lived out by Dr. Sartor: "The needs of the patient come first." This book is ultimately a story of that truth. It is part family memoir, part adventure, part past-as-prologue to our own time. As I read his story, I wondered how many people alive today owe their lives to Dr. Sartor and the 1,100 influenza patients he treated and cared for. Do they know the sacrifices that he made, that they might live and have families of their own today?

History records that Dr. Sartor visited Mayo Clinic but did not practice on our staff. Selfishly, I wish he had. I would have been privileged to know him and work alongside him. He clearly lived out the highest ideals of what each of us who practices at Mayo Clinic aspires to. Perhaps most importantly, Dr. Sartor discovered what many of us as seasoned clinicians learn — that the most important thing we ever do as physicians is to give hope and compassion to the sick. It is what most heals the human body and soul.

So, I invite you to read, imagine and meditate on Dr. Sartor's story, and particularly consider what made him such a heroic physician. Some of this, I fear, we have lost, but this book reminds us of the good, of the past, of what is really important when life and its circumstances demand of us what we were not prepared for. May we aspire to do as well in our pandemic as he did during his.

Gregory A. Poland, M.D.

Mary Lowell Leary Emeritus Professor of Medicine, Infectious Disease and
Molecular Pharmacology and Experimental Therapeutics
Director, Mayo Clinic Vaccine Research Group
Distinguished Investigator of Mayo Clinic

Dr. Sartor and Mayo Clinic

Collaboration and Inspiration

TEAMWORK IS THE HALLMARK OF MAYO CLINIC. The story of Dr. Pierre Sartor provides a unique perspective on this enduring value.

His practice in rural Iowa, which spanned the first half of the 20th century, illustrates a key aspect of Mayo's mission and culture: respectful collaboration with referring physicians and other health care providers.

This commitment is expressed in the Mayo Clinic Model of Care, a statement of attributes that have defined Mayo across the arc of our institutional history, guiding our work today and into the future. The Mayo Clinic Model of Care is so important as to be literally carved in stone. You will find its full text, including the following words, on the marble wall of our museum and welcome center, Mayo Clinic Heritage Hall:

RESPECT FOR THE PATIENT, FAMILY AND THE PATIENT'S REFERRING PHYSICIAN

As colleagues, patients and friends, the Sartor family has a relationship with Mayo Clinic that spans more than a century.

On February 3, 1908, Pierre Sartor (seventh from top) signed the Surgeons Register of Saint Marys Hospital when he visited the Mayo brothers.

Name	Richmond, Va.
Feb 3rd 1908 Coleman Motley	
D. J. Thing	Willow City No. Dak.
C. A. Call	Greeley Colo
J. T. Reid.	Iola Kans.
H. M. Schaffer	Canton O
W T Phelps	Martinsville Ill
Pierre Sartor	Bancroft Ia.
J. G. Millspaugh	Little Falls, Minn
B. McConlon	Owatonna Minn
A. L. Cunningham	Oakland California
H. R. Gibson	Richmond Ky.
S. W. Brown	Tacoma Wn
V. J. Herald	Warrens Wis
Feb 10. F. L. Larimore	Mt Vernon Ill
W. F. Church	Greeley Colo.
C R Phelps	Casey Ill
H C wright	Che
F. W. Robbins	Dierah
Willard Bartlett	St. Louis (7+ trip)
Oplus Luedeking	St. Louis, Mo.
Carl A. Hamilton	Litchfield Minn.

This book focuses on the crucible experience of the 1918-1919 influenza pandemic, from an unpublished memoir by Dr. Sartor titled "Thrills of my life — specifically my 'Flu Life.'"

Like Dr. William Worrall Mayo, who founded our medical practice, Dr. Sartor was an immigrant — short of stature, towering in his commitment to excellence on behalf of patients. Like Mother Alfred Moes, who founded Saint Marys Hospital as Dr. Mayo's partner in healing, Dr. Sartor was a native of Luxembourg and exhibited many of the tenacious qualities that Mother Alfred described as "our faith and hope and energy."

Dr. Sartor was a few years younger than Dr. Mayo's surgeon-sons, Drs. William J. and Charles H. Mayo, and was one of many physicians who referred patients to them for specialized care. With his European education and practical experience in community medicine, Dr. Sartor would have relished the intellectual stimulation of being with peers from throughout the United States and abroad who gathered in Rochester, Minnesota, to observe surgery and exchange ideas.

In the early 1900s, visiting physicians like Dr. Sartor called these informal educational sessions "the Mayos' clinic," which referred to a hospital-based teaching event. That phrase was picked up by the railroads as they brought increasing numbers of patients to Rochester, and it entered the mass media that reported on the brothers' distinctive model of medical care. In 1914, the words were carved above the door of the first building that was designed for our practice. Dr. Sartor, therefore, was part of the generation of physicians who gave us our name: Mayo Clinic.

The subtitle of this book refers to journeys of a country doctor and highlights another Mayo Clinic connection to Dr. Sartor. *When Winter Came* is the story of a physician's personal and professional development. As a teaching institution, Mayo knows the importance of helping medical professionals find the path that will help them flourish. Decisions about which specialty to pursue and where to practice shape a physician's career satisfaction and productivity — with the ultimate beneficiaries being patients who receive high-quality care.

Dr. Sartor undertook many journeys in his life: geographic, medical and spiritual. Helped and inspired by others, he paid it forward through the care he provided to patients and the example he set for his son Guido to become a physician. While much has changed since Dr. Sartor's time, the events that helped form his character offer perspective today.

Humor was a saving grace for Dr. Sartor. He enjoyed describing the time he was roused from sleep and summoned to the telephone. He listened to the patient, gave helpful advice and could not forbear asking at the end of their conversation: *Why, why do you always call me at night?*

Whereupon the patient helpfully explained: *But, Doctor, you're so busy during the day!*

As the granddaughter of Pierre Sartor and author of this book, Mary Beth Sartor Obermeyer brings unique family insights to the story. As a journalist who has published three previous books, she draws upon her grandfather's handwritten memoir, letters and articles written about him and her years of absorbing family stories, all of which are augmented with research and creative expression. Information about Mayo Clinic provides context to her story of a rural physician who partnered with a destination medical center.

Through a robust collaboration, this book was produced during the COVID-19 era. This reminded us that although history does not repeat itself, it does come in cycles. While COVID and the influenza pandemic stretched across multiple calendar years, the season of winter is an apt metaphor for those who seek to do the best of things in the worst of times.

Dr. Will Mayo, whom Dr. Sartor admired, wrote: "The glory of medicine is that it is constantly moving forward, that there is always more to learn." Today we have many more resources than were available to Dr. Sartor when he described how influenza "spread like wildfire on wild prairie land."

But we in the 21st century would do well to reflect upon the scenes in this book that show Pierre Sartor at his best: He is sitting with a patient long into the night by the glow of a kerosene lamp. He is using innovative, results-based methods, making observations that will improve his service to other patients in the future. And he is also entirely present with the desperately ill person before him. Along with the contents of his doctor's bag, he offers the patient a warm touch, gentle conversation — and prayer. It is *caring* in the full and best sense of the word.

As one of Pierre's friends wrote: "All in all, the community of Titonka knows that Doctor Sartor is practicing among them to serve them. They are appreciatively aware of the fact that he will always go to any end to help them. For that, they love him."

From his writings and the stories that his granddaughter shares, we know Dr. Sartor did not have an elaborate philosophy of life. *Nothing easy*, he would say. *But keep agoing, keep agoing.*

That is good advice for us all, medical professionals and patients alike. Because when winter comes, you want a doctor like Pierre Sartor.

Matthew D. Dacy, M.A.
Director, Mayo Clinic Heritage Hall and Co-Chair, Mayo Clinic Heritage Days
Assistant Professor of History of Medicine

Christopher J. Boes, M.D.
Professor of Neurology and History of Medicine
Medical Director, W. Bruce Fye Center for the History of Medicine at Mayo Clinic

Pierre joined physicians from throughout the United States and around the world who gathered to observe the Mayo brothers in surgery. They wore colored ribbons to identify themselves as guests.

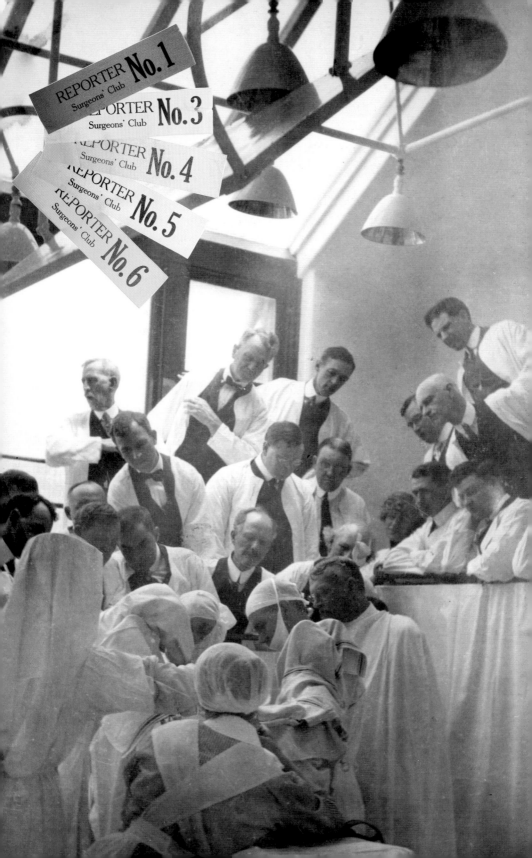

REPORTER No. 1
Surgeons' Club

REPORTER No. 3
Surgeons' Club

REPORTER No. 4
Surgeons' Club

REPORTER No. 5
Surgeons' Club

REPORTER No. 6
Surgeons' Club

Pierre Sartor — A Timeline

1871 (August 23) — Pierre was born in Berbourg, Luxembourg.

1883-1893 — Following the death of his mother, Catherine, Pierre lived in Esch-sur-Alzette for treatment of an ear condition. He then lived in Echternach and Luxembourg City while continuing his studies.

1893 — Pierre immigrated to the United States.

1893-1896 — Pierre attended Bennett Medical College in Chicago, Illinois, where he earned an M.D. degree.

1896 — Pierre visited Bancroft, Iowa, where he considered establishing his medical practice, but returned to Chicago to fill a need upon the death of a local physician.

1896-1901 — Pierre practiced in Chicago and undertook specialty training.

1898 (October 20) — Pierre married Mary Winandy.

1901 — Pierre and Mary moved their family to Bancroft, Iowa. They eventually had six children. As part of his medical practice, Pierre established a collaboration with Mayo Clinic that extended throughout his career.

1918 — Pierre moved his family to Titonka, Iowa, coinciding with the onset of the influenza pandemic.

1918-1919 — Pierre cared for people in Titonka and the surrounding region during the influenza pandemic. On many occasions, his 12-year-old son, Guido, drove him in a Model T Ford or sleigh to see patients.

1936 — Guido graduated from medical school at the University of Iowa. He subsequently received specialty training and practiced in Chicago.

1941 — Guido and his wife, Luella, moved to Mason City, Iowa, where he practiced and where they lived with their four children, including Mary Beth, the author of this book. Guido also collaborated with Mayo Clinic throughout his career.

1940-1950s — The author grew up hearing stories from and about her grandfather, Pierre Sartor.

1946 — Pierre was honored for serving as a physician for 50 years. He missed the celebration because he was busy attending a patient.

1953 — Pierre was named General Practitioner of the Year by the Iowa State Medical Society. (He also missed the meeting that nominated him for this award because he was caring for a patient.) Pierre wrote his memoir about the influenza pandemic and delivered it as a speech on multiple occasions. During the celebration of his 82nd birthday, he was reunited with a patient he first met as a child during the influenza pandemic.

1958 — Pierre died (August 5), shortly before his 87th birthday. Mary died (November 1) shortly after her 79th birthday and their 60th wedding anniversary.

2001 — The author received a lockbox with documents and artifacts from her father, Dr. Guido Sartor, and grandfather, Dr. Pierre Sartor. The contents of the lockbox, along with stories that she had heard over many years and her own research and creative reflections, form the basis of this book.

2004 (February 23) — Guido Sartor died, nine years to the day after his wife, Luella.

2020-2022 — The worldwide outbreak of COVID-19 prompted renewed interest in the influenza pandemic of 1918-1919.

2023 — Pierre's life story was published in collaboration with Mayo Clinic.

Table of Contents

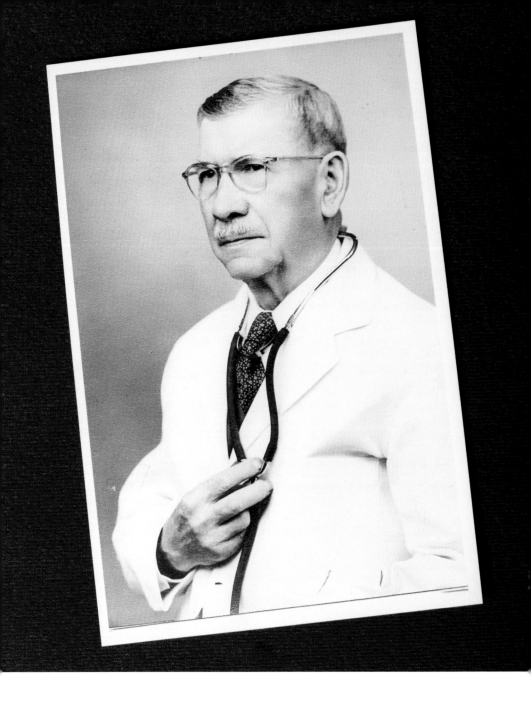

*Pierre Sartor was a beloved doctor who served his patients and collab-
orated with Mayo Clinic. The map shows Bancroft and Titonka, Iowa,
where Pierre practiced, along with other Midwestern sites in this story.*

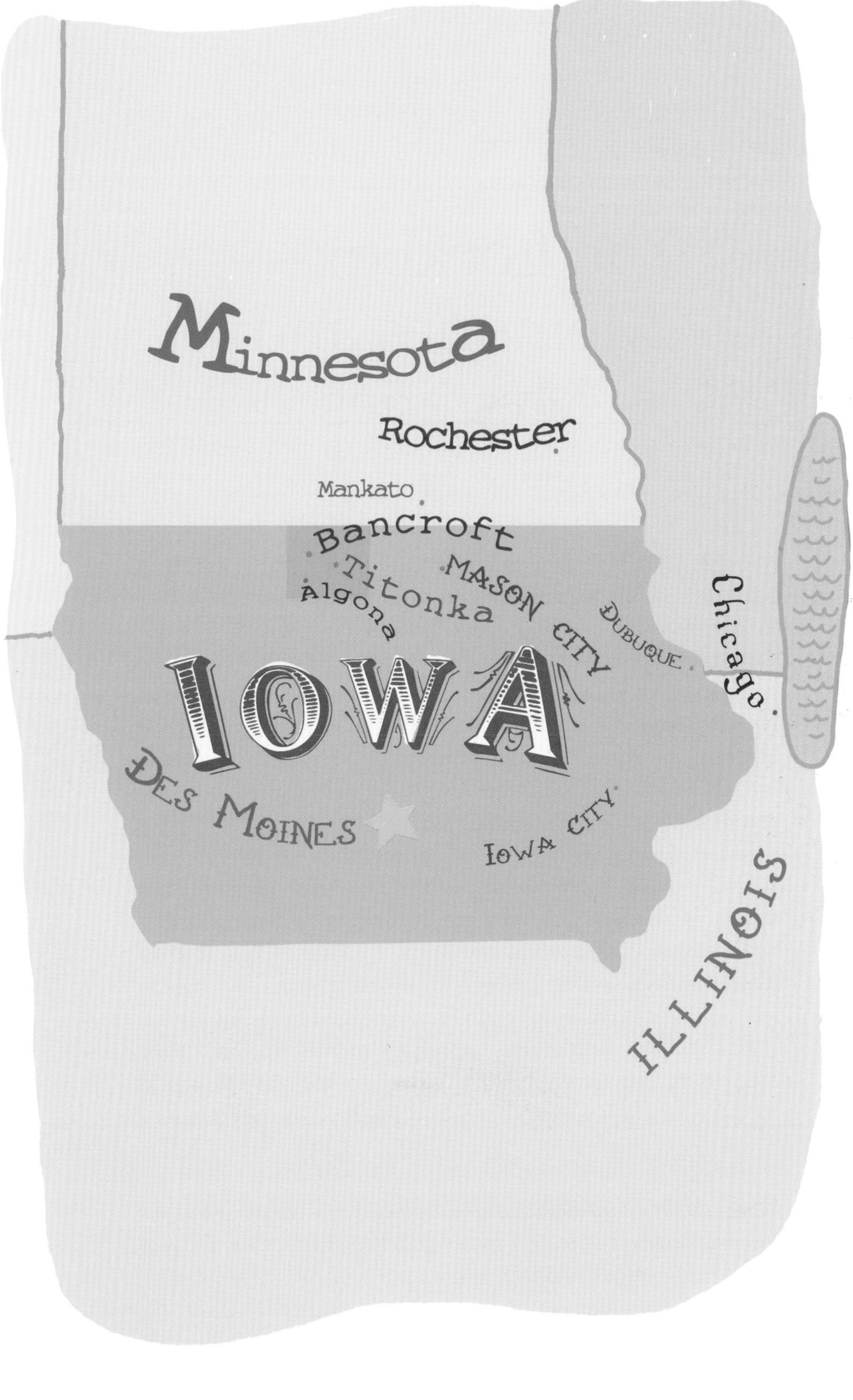
Minnesota
Rochester
Mankato
Bancroft
Titonka
Algona
MASON CITY
DUBUQUE
Chicago
IOWA
DES MOINES
IOWA CITY
ILLINOIS

The Lockbox — Memories and Mysteries

MY GRANDFATHER, DR. PIERRE SARTOR, WROTE A MEMOIR of his experiences during the winter of 1918. The influenza pandemic that year ravaged the world, but for Grandpa it was a battle to save his friends and neighbors in the small town of Titonka, located in north-central Iowa, and others who lived in the hamlets and on farms nearby. Throughout much of the crisis, Grandpa was the sole physician, working with a network of dedicated volunteers he recruited from the community and even from his own family.

Grandpa read his memoir as a speech that he delivered on several occasions, decades after the pandemic. Today, more than a century has passed since the events he described. His handwritten pages are at my home in Minneapolis. I keep them right where they've been for so many years — between leather covers and wrapped in string, nestled in his lockbox.

That lockbox, containing Grandpa's manuscript and other artifacts of our family history, passed to his son Dr. Guido Sartor — my father — and eventually to me. My first memory

When author Mary Beth Sartor Obermeyer was growing up, she imagined a world of secrets in her grandfather's lockbox. Decades later, the tales began to emerge.

of it dates to the mid-1940s when I was little, stalling bedtime, peeking into my father's den at our home in Mason City, Iowa, where I grew up. Likely as not, Grandpa, who often visited us, was bent over that very box.

Sometimes, if I was lucky, Grandpa would spy me and pull me to his lap. He'd switch on my father's reel-to-reel tape recorder, put the big silver microphone before us and begin to tell a story. Not a fairy tale, no. His stories were real — and they were magical.

Once upon a time, Grandpa Pierre would begin, *I sailed across the ocean with my lockbox on a tramp steamer.* The journey was dangerous, but Grandpa and his box survived, making the trip from his homeland in Luxembourg to America.

Even sitting on his lap, I couldn't see everything inside the box that held his memories. But I could imagine. Of one thing I was sure: That box overflowed with treasures . . . pebbles . . . bird wings . . . clouds! I was four.

Imagine then, Christmas Day in 2001, as the thermometer neared zero — my father, Guido, nearing 100 — when that very lockbox was placed into my hands. It was a simple transfer, after Mass, in the parking lot of Holy Family Catholic Church in Mason City. The time had come in our family to pass things around. At least the important things. And I was to copy the contents of the lockbox for my sisters, Celeste and Julie, and my brother, Bob.

As the newest caretaker of the box, once again I felt its aura, stirring memories from years before.

That night, my husband, Tom, a Twin Cities architect, and I made our slow drive home, two hours through ice and fog. When we arrived, I clutched the box and pushed open my front door. And I would like to say that I settled by the fireplace with a cider and a quilt and delved right into the mysteries of the lockbox. But, no, I was tired. I opened it, but all I could see was a stack of papers. I glanced at some of them, then closed the lid and went to bed.

Another day, soon after, I put the lockbox on a shelf. It would keep.

My father died in 2004. Though I've been a "Luxie," an enthusiast for Luxembourg, for as long as I can remember, his passing intensified my interest in our homeland. I have visited twice. The first time was in 1979 with Tom and a group of his architecture students. The second time was in 2019, five years after Tom's death, when I became a dual citizen of the United States and Luxembourg. Generations of my family have made multiple trips to Luxembourg since World War II, and more than a dozen of us have become or are in the process of becoming dual citizens. From favorite recipes to figures of speech in our conversation, the roots run deep.

Luxembourg is a tiny country — less than 1,000 square miles, one of the smallest sovereign states in the world — with castles and farms, hedgehogs and broom flowers. Surrounded by France, Belgium and Germany, it includes dense forests, lush river valleys and craggy cliffs. A bird — a stonechat — warbles *chat-chat*.

My heightened interest in our family roots prompted a return to the lockbox. One day I took it down from the shelf and creaked it open. I examined each document, gently lifting, sifting. Ribbons of reel-to-reel tape became caught up in my fingers. Medical papers from my grandfather and father were in there. Letters and yellowed newspapers curled and broke, brittle, coming apart at the folds.

But what I found next has captivated me from that day onward and brings me to share this story with you. An inked title caught the light: *"Thrills of my life — specifically my 'Flu Life.'"*

I had discovered my grandfather's first-person account of the great influenza pandemic of 1918-1919.

Pierre's efforts during that muddy, miserable winter were a staple of conversation when I was growing up. It was said in family discussions that Grandpa treated more than 1,000 patients with remarkably few deaths, even though no one at the time knew how influenza spreads and despite the lack of effective medications.

As I got older, I wondered if this was the kind of hyperbole that can slip into a family's collective memory — but as I read the manuscript that day, these words leaped out in my grand-father's Old World penmanship:

> *Right here let me say, that in 5 months and a half I lost only 5 flu victims out of a total about eleven hundred cases bed-fast, not light perambulatory cases counted even.*

His accomplishment was startling, extraordinary. While conducting research for this book, I found Pierre's statement repeated in a statewide medical publication and in interviews that he gave — at a time when many people who experienced the pandemic were alive to corroborate his account.

How did he do it? What was his plan? This was something to be explored — and shared.

I quickly did the math. I was 17 when Pierre died in 1958, old enough to have gained a firsthand appreciation of what a unique man he was. I loved listening to our family stories, paying closer attention, I now realize, than youngsters typically do when their elders reminisce. My mother, Luella, used to say I was taking inventory.

During the summer after fifth grade, the risk of another pandemic — polio — kept me indoors while a newspaper reporter conducted an extensive interview with Grandpa. With a wink to me, Grandpa told the reporter he would begin his story when he was 11 years old — that was my age! On that afternoon — and now, even more so — I felt him reaching out to me in a special way. I was also pleasantly aware that the journalist who wrote about Grandpa was a woman.

In my career, I have been a technical writer and editor. I've published three books. One was a finalist for the Midwest Book Award.

I could write his story!

I had the mother lode of documentation. Pierre received

In the 1940s and '50s, author Mary Beth Sartor Obermeyer enjoyed spending time with her grandparents, Dr. Pierre and Mary Sartor, and often visited their home in Titonka, Iowa.

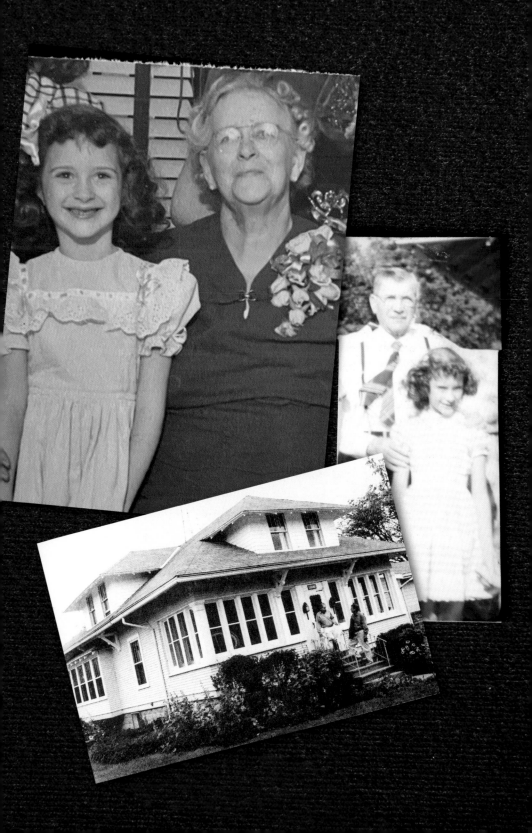

many professional honors, and articles about him have been preserved in family scrapbooks. Letters and photos — even clothing such as Pierre's elegant frock coat and his first child's baptismal gown, made of delicate lace imported from France — have survived. The archives of the local newspaper, *Titonka Topic*, provide a glimpse into the daily life in the close-knit community that Pierre served for 40 years.

Seemingly random events took on new meaning: At my father's estate sale, I chose a marble penholder attached to a framed image of the Madonna, not realizing what it was, because the pen was missing. Later, I discovered that Grandpa used that same inkstand during the time of the pandemic.

I've got this.

My grandfather's life was a journey, and I've found that writing a book is an undertaking of its own. You meet many people along the way and sometimes you find yourself heading in unexpected directions before reaching the destination.

Early on, I shared this project with several physicians, including my neighbor, Dr. Kristine Ensrud. They asked questions, not technical at all, just those benign queries that insightful physicians use to discern important facts — in this case, how my grandfather could keep so many patients alive when death was all around. They asked what Dr. Sartor did. In response, I summarized Grandpa's memoir.

Pierre's prescription for fighting the flu was a blend of head and heart: isolating the ill and training family members to be caregivers, augmented by strict hygiene, compassion, music — and prayer.

Their conclusion? I didn't see it coming: *cutting edge* and *ahead of his time*. Grandpa was spot-on accurate in using the knowledge of his day, they said; moreover, he systematically applied precepts that were not standard in the medical profession until years later. Dr. Ensrud picked up on the fact that Pierre could never have achieved such results by himself. The townspeople had to believe — and work cooperatively with Pierre and each other, both as patients and as volunteer caregivers.

Then again, Grandpa did have charisma. People were drawn to him for his skill, compassion and calm good judgment, even when life and death were in the balance.

In researching and writing about my grandfather, I came to realize that his outer story, dramatic and well documented as it is, cloaks an equally compelling inner story. I could not fully understand why Pierre took the path he did until I talked to David Brooks when he came to Minneapolis soon after writing *The Road to Character*.

The qualities of character that Brooks described made me think of Grandpa:

> *You don't ask, What do I want from life? You ask a different set of questions: What does life want from me? What are my circumstances calling me to do? In this scheme of things we don't create our lives; we are summoned by life.*

After graduating from medical school, Pierre established a successful practice in Chicago. He achieved further status through marriage: Mary Winandy, the love of his life, came from a background of financial prosperity and social prominence. But one day Pierre moved his young family from their affluent circle to a town on the Iowa prairie. In the spring of 1918, at the start of the influenza pandemic, he uprooted his family again and relocated to an even smaller town in Iowa, which had no doctor of its own. Pierre explained both moves with the simple words, *I am needed*.

The lockbox continued to reveal its treasures. I found an article about Mayo Clinic to which my grandfather had added in his own handwriting, "The Mayo Miracle." I had heard of Mayo Clinic all my life; Grandpa and my father often referred patients there. As physicians, they considered Mayo to be their partner for difficult cases. Pierre and Guido enjoyed friendships with colleagues on the Mayo Clinic staff and shared important life experiences with the Mayo family. The *Titonka Topic* faithfully chronicled over the course of many years when townsfolk went "to Mayos" for consultation or surgery.

My own introduction to Mayo Clinic was through another

type of referral. As I researched publishers for this book, my friend David Unowsky, with whom I've collaborated on literary projects for more than 30 years, suggested Mayo. Conversations began during the COVID-19 pandemic, which gave fresh perspective to my grandfather's work in 1918. Mayo Clinic affirmed Pierre's methods.

Collaboration with Mayo Clinic revealed key points of connection, which are woven into the narrative. The "aha" moment came when the Mayo team showed me Pierre Sartor's signature as one of the earliest names in the clinic's guestbook of visiting physicians, dated February 3, 1908. At the other end of the time spectrum, our family archive contains a letter that a doctor at Mayo Clinic wrote to my father more than 70 years after Pierre's first visit. This book, therefore, continues a close, ongoing relationship between my family and Mayo Clinic that has thrived for more than a century. At its deepest level, shared values link Mayo Clinic in Rochester, Minnesota, and Dr. Pierre Sartor in Titonka, Iowa.

Pierre said he would not die wealthy. And he was right — many times, his patients paid him in livestock and crops. But, by his own measure, did he succeed? As he would say: *Some days were good; some days not so good. But I kept agoing, kept agoing, and if that isn't a good life, I don't know what is.*

This positive and purposeful outlook sustained Pierre through long, eventful years, including what he called the "Thrills of my life" — the influenza pandemic.

I want to share my grandfather's life with you as a story. It's based upon his memoir and the oft-told tales I have heard from the family, as well as my research and interpretations — along with some questions yet to be answered.

Growing up, I heard my grandfather tell these stories in person and on the tape recordings that my father made of Pierre reminiscencing. My father had a large collection of those tapes and he played them over and over again. At our house in Mason City, Daddy's den was just below my second-floor bedroom. He usually played the tapes after my brother, sisters and I went to bed; on many a night, Grandpa's voice on a tape recording lulled me to sleep. Today, more than 60 years after Pierre died, I can hear the inimitable click and slursh of his voice: words and accents that reflected his knowledge of German, French, English and Luxembourgish, the dialect of Luxembourg — with some terms in Latin thrown in for good measure. Pierre's stories formed the background of my life.

Even before I began working on this book, I wrote standalone scenes that depict key moments in our family history. I asked my father to read them, and they met his stringent standards for accuracy. A picture of me showing him some writing samples is one of my most "liked" photos on Facebook. You might think of this book as a collection of those scenes, like squares in a quilt, stitched together through the creative process.

Pierre's story will take us to certain times and places. But every family has its own version of the lockbox: a collection of memories and objects passed down through the years, continually enriched by new people and experiences.

I hope Pierre and the others you will meet become friendly companions as you pursue dreams of your own amid the challenges and blessings of life.

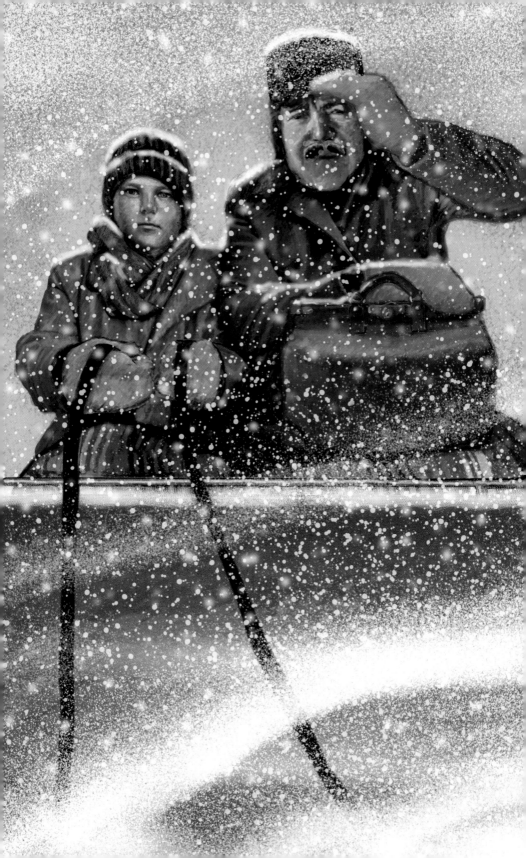

CHAPTER 1

Setting Forth

The Iowa Prairie
February 3, 1919 — Morning

OVERNIGHT, GUSTS OF COLD AIR had skittered along the storm windows, leaving a thick coat of white frosting on all three sides of the porch. As the local newspaper would report: "Monday morning when we awoke all of north Iowa was in the throes of a fierce blizzard. Snow was piled up several feet deep in places on Main Street."

The heavy, new-fallen snow was a change: So far, this winter had been unusually mild, murky with mud. From inside his snug house, Dr. Pierre Sartor adjusted the flaps of his hat and headed out the door.

The front steps were slippery. The snow-over-slush had turned to ice, bringing more difficulties to a day already filled with challenges.

Pierre's colleague Dr. N.D. Ray in the nearby town of Woden had taken ill and Pierre had to travel beyond his own familiar

Despite an early morning blizzard, Pierre and his son Guido were determined to see his patients, many of whom lived on isolated farms deep in the Iowa prairie.

territory to see Dr. Ray's rural patients; they could not wait for better weather. Pierre later wrote that one young mother "came down with the flu and a severe pneumonia complication." The stakes were high for her and many others. Unlike the flu of previous years, what was going around in this winter of 1918-1919 struck young adults with special virulence. The combination of influenza and pneumonia was often lethal.

Pierre had been to see the mother, along with several other patients under Dr. Ray's care, the day before. He contemplated today's journey — more than 15 miles round trip, pulled by horses over rutted roads made worse by the ice and snow — with grim determination.

A silver sky nipped at the earth. Low-hung clouds seemed trapped in the tips of fleecy evergreens. Soon snowmen would fill the yards in Titonka, the small Iowa town where he had settled his family a few months before. Already, it felt like home.

Unfortunately, real people would not be about. The children who made the snowmen would not play long outside. They would soon be redirected indoors.

Titonka was in quarantine.

Pierre straddled the steps, going down one at a time, and steadied his way to the street. Just getting to Dr. Ray's patients — now, his patients — was an arduous undertaking. The horses and sleigh waiting in front of his house would take him on the first leg of the journey, from Titonka toward Woden. At a rendezvous point three miles outside Woden, a wagon and a fresh team of horses would be ready to take him on the final part of the trip, going deep into the Iowa prairie.

Pierre kicked the runner of the sleigh to chuck heavy snow from his boot. He hoisted himself up and into the sleigh, and then waited. Pierre would not make this difficult trip alone. He looked around for his driver — the steady, reliable companion who not only ensured his safe arrival at the isolated homes of people stricken with life-threatening illness but also put himself in harm's way to assist Pierre, effectively carrying out the doctor's unique methods of treatment, which were keeping so many patients alive.

Pierre's driver was Guido, his 12-year-old son.

At that moment, Guido had priorities of his own. He was finishing breakfast. Warm milk and *sterzelen*, a buckwheat breakfast cake, traditional to Luxembourg and made with love by his mother, Pierre's wife, Mary, would provide the energy that their elder son needed this day.

Pierre absently squeezed his mustache, up to down, center to edge. He dipped his chin under his scarf to blot. He stilled himself, but his insides churned.

It was almost a year since the influenza began. The flu ebbed and flowed at first, but since last fall it had consumed their lives. Pierre was in his fifth month of fighting the flu nonstop. Drained at the end of long days and burdened with his patients' anxiety, Pierre used one of his characteristic colloquial phrases, "My heart break," with increasing frequency.

The cold wind blew through his heart. This ill mother might be the start of . . . a further outbreak? He didn't know. Pierre was just starting to serve the area around Woden. While he had established protocols to limit the spread of influenza in and around Titonka — and, for the most part, secured people's co-operation, which resulted in many lives being saved — conditions in his new territory were different. In many respects, he was starting over, trying to introduce unfamiliar methods to people he didn't know as the disease raged among them.

Upon seeing the mother the day before, Pierre made a key observation. It was not the woman's clinical condition that riveted him. He would devote knowledge and skills to care for her, and he was confident that she would accept the treatment he offered. No, what worried Pierre most was the fact that his patient held her toddler daughter close, snug in bed together.

The scene, so natural and comforting in times of good health, was a deadly risk to the child:

> One of my rules strictly enforced if possible was 'isolation' no 2 patients in any one room, and much less in one bed.

Before Pierre left his patient's home, he clamped a clothespin inside the mother's bedsheet to isolate her within the covers.

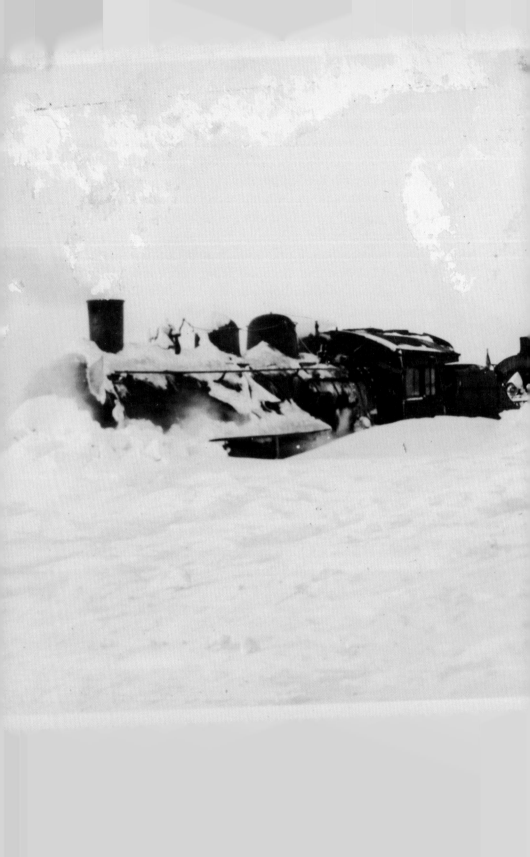

He removed the young daughter, calmed her against his chest and took her to the next room to check her. Thank the good Lord, the child appeared fine.

Pierre made plans for another family to take the child overnight, but he left before that happened. A sense of regret gnawed at him. Looking back, he should have sent the toddler with Guido to a nearby barn, to wait for the transfer to a healthy family's home; at least then he would be sure it had been done.

Another phrase Pierre used often came readily to mind: "Nothing easy."

If the mother died, the child would end up living with relatives. Pierre had lost his mother at a young age and his life took an entirely new direction from that wrenching experience. And if the child died . . . Pierre knew there was no greater anguish for a parent. Deep within, Pierre felt worries for his own son Anthony, Guido's younger brother, who was about the age of the little girl in Woden. Anthony had been frail since birth and showed no sign of improving.

The family in Woden . . . Had the mother listened? Was the child in a safe place?

A sense of mission drove Pierre. It's what had brought him to Titonka in the first place, by coincidence almost a year earlier, just as the influenza pandemic was beginning. The town of approximately 350 people — about 50 miles west of Mason City, Iowa, and 75 miles south of Mankato, Minnesota — was in dire straits, its only doctor recently departed to serve in the Great War.

Pierre waited. His anxiety grew into frustration.

At long last, Mary came onto the porch, followed by most of their children — tumbling out of the house, swooshing around her skirts with a scoot and a slide. It was the family's early

This photo from the Sartor family collection shows a winter storm in rural Iowa. These are the same conditions that Pierre and Guido encountered when they traveled together.

morning ritual, which provided the youngsters a brief time of fresh air amid the dreary quarantine of winter.

They ran to the porch, so they could look out into the yard. Pierre and Mary had six children, and five of them appeared: May, age 19; Magdalene, 16; Mercedes, 10; Alice, 6; and Anthony, 4. Oh, the snow! With schools closed for quarantine, they were in a commotion.

Arms-a-windmill, Mary moved across the porch, attending each child. This was one of the days Mary would say to her brood, *Bundle up! You may run in the garden*. The Sartor family lived on two double lots: half for their house and yard with an equivalent space alongside for the garden. Mary's dried flowers stood proud in the garden. Stalks poked through the fresh snow, etched as lace. They made a wonderland of a maze.

Mary's idea of using the garden as a maze probably came from a novel she read to her children. *The Secret Garden* by Frances Hodgson Burnett told how a girl named Mary Lennox lost her parents in an epidemic of cholera. Sent to live with her uncle, Mary discovers a garden that brings her joy and hope. The garden also becomes a place where Colin, her sickly cousin, is restored to health.

Mary waved to Pierre as she released their children into the yard; his St. Mary she was. Pierre knew that when Mary got their children chasing in the garden, she was boosting their spirits, dispensing her own kind of medicine.

Throughout the winter, Mary hid a surprise for her children to discover each day they romped in the garden. It might be a holy card with a saint's name on one side and a prayer on the other — or it might be a cookie or other homemade treat. Pierre smiled. With any luck, it would take the children a long, delightful time to find today's treasure. All the while, Mary would get a drawn-out moment for herself, with a glass of sun tea by the stove. Pierre knew his wife's heart must race sometimes, for need of peace, some space.

Families were challenged in the winter of 1918-1919. Children on the Iowa prairie were used to living free-range. The flu forced them indoors. They were protected, but this quarantine choked.

Finally — Pierre enjoyed watching his children, but he needed his older son to get the day's work started, and Guido was typically the last to show up. Today again he earned his nickname, Swifty Sartor, arriving just as Pierre reached the end of his patience. As Guido dashed across the porch, Mary wrapped a sweater about his neck, secure. She yanked his jacket right, pulling it over his knickers.

The boy hugged his mother and spun on, stomping down the front steps. He hopped into the sleigh with glass jars under his arm — pickled pig feet for lunch and hocks of hog, which he and his father would share on what they anticipated would be a long day. Pierre had a buffalo robe over his lap and lifted it for Guido to come under as well. Pierre pushed a giant safety pin through the robe to hold them both tight and warm.

Pierre had made Guido his driver on and off all winter as they traveled to widely scattered houses and farms. For Pierre, it was a chance to rest. For Guido, it was the experience of a lifetime.

At 12 years of age, Guido was an accomplished driver, not only of horses but at the wheel of his family's Model T Ford as well. Automobiles were still a novelty; the few regulations that were on the books were lightly enforced in rural America. Guido loved driving the car and his penchant for speed caused memorable mishaps. On this day, however, they would travel by sleigh — a more reliable method given the weather, but there was no windshield to protect them.

Showing a man's confidence and skill, Guido took the reins. With a flip of his wrist, he urged the horses forward. As the sleigh lurched to a start, Pierre hoped the ruts they would find in the open country ahead had been dragged. Hardened mud could be treacherous.

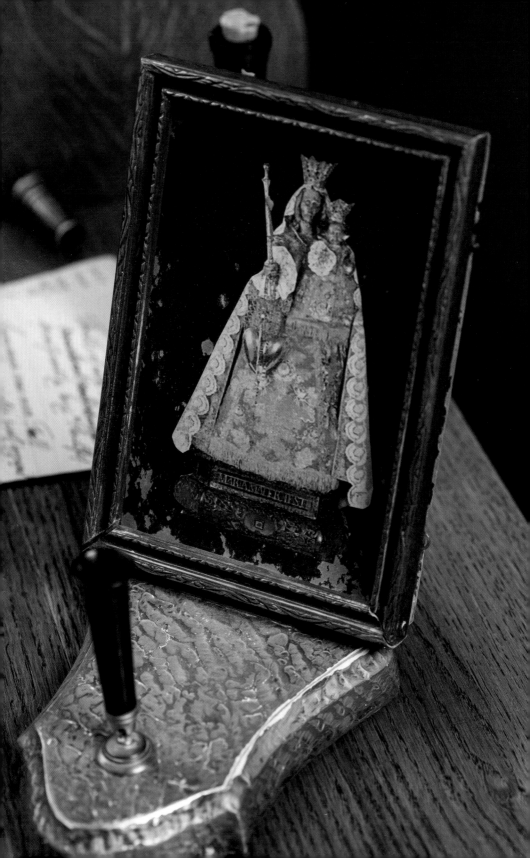

CHAPTER 2

"...if you make that one well..."

The Iowa Prairie
February 3, 1919 — Late Afternoon and Evening

PIERRE NUDGED GUIDO. It was his reminder: *Boy, don't lick your lips!* Each morning, they slathered glycerin over their faces as protection from the elements. It was a form of sugar. Tempted to lick, Iowa kids got raw skin, upper lips to the nose, in winter.

Making their way through Titonka, they passed homes and businesses that were eerily quiet. Many of the town's men were serving in the military, and quarantine muted the sounds of women and children. There would be no sidewalk conversations, no courtesies, no casual "How d'ye do?" to Pierre's neighbors and patients.

On this day, for Pierre, there would be no nodding off either, as was his wont when he craved rest. Pierre would keep lookout as Guido drove the horses.

Pierre used this inkstand to record his experiences during the 1918 pandemic. Reflecting his strong faith, the inkstand includes an image of Our Lady of Luxembourg — "Comforter of the Afflicted."

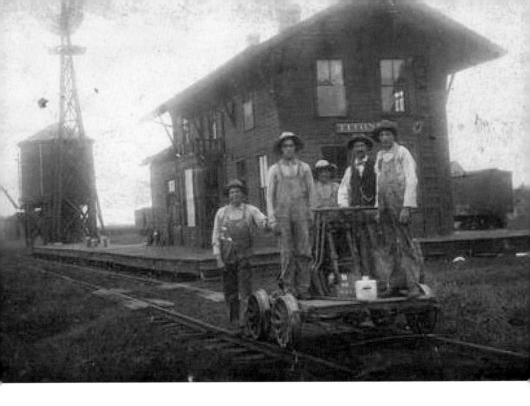

As for Guido? He relaxed a bit because he could, while Pa was fresh. It might even have been fun for a while, father and son together. Soon they left town and were in the open countryside. They took turns spitting — a bonding ritual for boys and men of all ages. It was a type of freedom that even thoroughly domesticated males enjoyed, something they could not do readily in mixed company. It also represented the lure of the outdoors because spittoons were banned in many businesses and private homes this flu season.

It was snowing steadily and now the wind picked up. Winter had come, and in force.

Pierre and Guido settled down, concentrating harder. The fences that marked the edge of the road — *Where were they?* And the ground beneath, it shivered and shook. Or so it seemed, coming from the rhythm of the ruts as the sleigh jolted along. They clutched the seat and tried not to bounce. The sleigh lurched, and Pierre had to press hard into Guido's young shoulder, just to stay a-right.

The horizon should have been there, but it was not. It was

gone, vanished into the sky. Pierre and Guido were nearly blinded by the swirling and drifting snow. They lost track of time and direction.

I remember my grandfather, when he told this story, saying he hoped Guido would not drive into the slough. Pronounced "slew," it is the main geographic feature of the area, the remains of a preglacial riverbed, a marshland that covered about 8,000 acres at that time and today is known as the Union Slough National Wildlife Refuge. Anyone who entered that bog in a blizzard was unlikely to come out alive. Grandpa was making a point about how utterly lost they were and how dangerous the situation was: The slough is due west of Titonka, while their intended destination was due east.

Pierre looked at his son and fought a rising sense of fear. Pierre's own father had frozen to death in just such a blizzard, back in Luxembourg, not long before.

It must have seemed an eternity, but at some point, the sound of a train whistle and the light of its headlight cut through the storm. I believe that although Pierre and Guido could not flag down the train as it passed, they were able to orient themselves by the direction it took. Following the tracks, they reached a station — but it was not the one where their wagon and fresh horses waited.

Pierre's resourcefulness and professional network now served them well. Since 1913, he had provided medical services to the Chicago, Rock Island and Pacific Railroad, known informally as the Rock Island Line. Pierre and Guido received a warm welcome from the crew.

Pierre arranged to borrow the railroad's hand-pumped cart, also called a "lorry," so he and Guido could ride the rails to where their wagon and fresh horses waited.

The railroad crewman and Pierre positioned the cart on the

Men at the Titonka railroad station gather around a hand-pumped lorry. Pierre and Guido used a similar vehicle to reach patients during the influenza pandemic.

rails. Guido tied the sleigh and its team of horses to a post; a neighbor would drive the hitch back to the stable.

Pierre gripped the bar of the cart and began to pump, slow to fast, propelling the cart along the railroad track. Furiously he had at it, working up a sweat in the bitter cold. He had to loop his doctor's bag by its handles around his wool-socked leg so it wouldn't fly away.

Guido hunched into a cocoon behind his father to protect his face from the wind, until it was his turn to pump. It was exhausting work in the brutal weather. And it was dangerous. Trains could appear suddenly, speeding forth with no awareness of pedestrians or vehicles like a lorry that might be using the railroad tracks to get from one place to another. By the time a train conductor saw anyone else on the tracks, it would be too late.

Then, suddenly, as if by magic, the blizzard stopped.

But the wind on the prairie — oh, how it can blow. It whipped everything to a freeze. And the snow turned to diamonds on the fields and the trees.

Finally, they reached the point where the horses and wagon were at the ready for the final leg of their journey.

They boarded the wagon and lumbered away over the icy, rutted ground. Although the blizzard had tapered off, the snow-covered ground and gray sky dimly lit by a weak sun caused near-whiteout conditions.

At last, they reached the patient's farm. After an exhausting trip, Pierre would now begin his medical duties for the day. Guido followed his father into the house like a shadow, comfort arriving in knickers and a face mask.

On his previous visit, Pierre had left clear instructions: *Move the child out of her mother's bed*. Pierre hoped the youngster was safe with neighbors down the road.

To his dismay, Pierre saw that the child had been moved — but only as far as "a little bed at the opposite corner of the room," as he later wrote. This hardly qualified as isolation — and, indeed, just as Pierre had feared, the girl was now desperately ill. Her mother was distraught. For Pierre, it must have been like a gut punch.

Although he had warned against exactly this outcome, and although he had put himself and his son through hours of toil just to get there, Pierre responded to the mother not with anger or frustration but with compassion. He understood parental bonds and the close ties of kin among the prairie families he served.

To extend his reach, Pierre had developed a network of volunteers who helped care for his patients and took in relatives who needed a place to stay. Two particularly dedicated volunteers are known to us from Pierre's memoir as "Tony" and "Tony's wife." It was to this couple that Pierre turned for help in caring for the mother and daughter. In essence, he gave these patients the best he had.

Pierre's methods worked and, even after such a hellish day, he and Guido returned to that farmhouse on multiple occasions.

Pierre's memoir describes "one day as the mother improved, some owing to the good care of Tony's wife." The fact that the mother was recovering, however, seems to have heightened her distress that by not heeding Pierre's call to separate herself from her daughter, she had endangered her child's life. Her daughter remained critically ill.

This led to one of the most significant and symbolic conversations in Pierre's life. Years later, he wrote: "Mother looked at me and said, pointing to the little girl, 'Doctor, if you make that one well again, you can ask of me anything you wish for.'"

Pierre thereupon made a wish, and yes, it did come true.

For all the exhaustion Pierre must have felt in that winter that seemed unending, closure would come on a blazing hot summer afternoon, decades later. As an elderly man, Pierre would experience renewal of life from this same farm family, much as he first discovered it during his own challenging childhood.

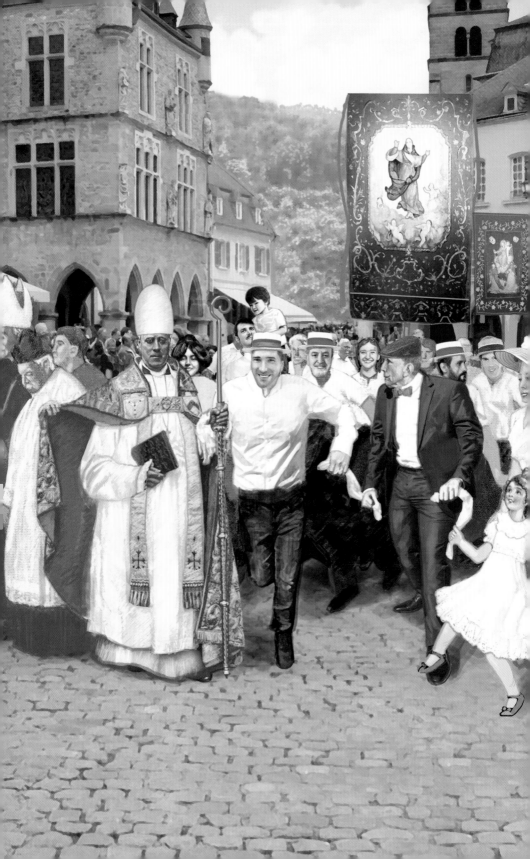

CHAPTER 3

Procession of the Faithful and a Mother's Funeral

Luxembourg
1882-1883

CHURCH BELLS WERE RINGING throughout the village of Berbourg. It was May 30, 1882: Whit Tuesday by the calendar of the Roman Catholic Church, which structured the year — and virtually all aspects of life — for 10-year-old Pierre Sartor, his family and everyone they knew.

The bells on this occasion proclaimed a holiday two days after Pentecost Sunday, which commemorates the descent of the Holy Spirit upon the apostles and disciples of Jesus. "Whit" is an ancient term that may be associated with the white robes worn by new members of the Catholic Church who are baptized at Pentecost or derived from "huit," the French word for "eight," representing the eight weeks that span Easter to Pentecost. With the arrival of spring, it was a time of renewal — of nature, and the human spirit.

As he struggled awake, Pierre had mixed feelings on this festive

"Please, God, a miracle." Carried amid the crowd of people who surged toward the church, Pierre prayed that his hearing impairment would be cured and that his mother would regain her strength.

day. He was excited because while people throughout Europe and beyond celebrate Whit Tuesday, Luxembourg has a one-of-a-kind event that takes place each year in the town of Echternach, less than eight miles from Pierre's home in Berbourg. Today, this event is recognized by the United Nations Educational, Scientific and Cultural Organization (UNESCO) as being part of the Intangible Cultural Heritage of Humanity.

It goes by the name of *Sprangprëssessioun*. To many people — in Pierre's time and today — it is known simply as the Hopping Procession. For centuries, throngs of church leaders, musicians and pilgrims have made their way through the medieval streets of Echternach, hopping and dancing in procession to the Abbey of St. Willibrord, where it is said the patron saint of Luxembourg dispenses miracles to the faithful, especially those who are afflicted with illness. In rows the people prance and parade. The German word describes it best — pronounced "schpring" — meaning to jump. For the Sartor family, this was a beloved annual tradition, the kind of ritual that grounds children, shapes the people they become.

At the same time, the ringing bells made Pierre wince. For as long as he could remember, Pierre suffered from pain in his ears. The gongs and clangs on this morning gave him a throbbing headache.

An idea began to form in Pierre's mind. The Hopping Procession had been part of his life for as long as he could remember. Now he began to associate it with his own condition. All those stories of old detailing miraculous cures — could it happen to him?

Pierre was steeped in the traditions of his people: customs and stories that predated or lived alongside Church teaching. In addition to devotion to St. Willibrord, the Hopping Procession was associated with the Legend of the Fiddler Thief:

> *Once upon a time in a small town there lived a man*
> *named Viedt. He was very poor and very crafty. But*
> *his luck ran out, and he was sentenced for his crimes.*
> *He was to be hanged. As was the custom, he was*
> *granted his last wish. He asked for a fiddle, and when*

he shouldered it, he began to play, Oh, how he played! Enchanted, the people began to skip and dance — such delightful chaos that when no one was watching the thief slipped away! He was saved forever!

Over the years, this story became part of the cultural legacy in Luxembourg so that dancing in the procession might serve as protection from plague — or as a way to be cured of other ailments.

This combination of faith and folklore gave Pierre extra enthusiasm for the special day. He was the baby, the youngest and frailest of all the children in his family, but he would go to the procession. This time, he felt added purpose and resolve. Even if his ears and head were thick with fluid, he knew the songs they would sing. The hymns throbbed, deep within his pain-filled ears.

Would he be strong enough to spring and hop with the others?

It could be said that Pierre was coddled, just a bit. While everyone had warming pans heated with coal under their beds, and heated bricks under the mattress to stay warm through the night, on each morning in fair weather, Pierre's mother, Catherine, took the extra effort to hang the boy's shirt on a hook in the courtyard of their home. Doing so bleached it pure white and warmed it in the sun. It would be there today.

Pierre's family lived in what we might call a row house. Their residence, with an elegant front door, stood next to a stable and barn, sharing walls with each.

Pierre got out of bed, struggled into his trousers and headed outdoors. He wanted his mother. He called to her.

"Pittchen!" she answered, her name of love, just for him. She spread her arms wide, held him close, blew softly into his ears, one after the other; it was a comfort. She helped Pierre as he wended his arms through the warm sleeves of the cotton shirt she had waiting for him. It helped soothe the rash that was so painful.

When Pierre was flush with fever, his mother held him close. Why was his skin warm and prickly while hers was cool and smooth? He did not know. The contrast was confusing. But surely, he believed, he would be all right as long as his mother took care of him.

Pierre always heard his mother best. Other people, he could not hear so well. Pierre figured he was like an ox. He heard coos or shouts — what people intended, although not always the specific words they used. But he always knew what his mother was saying to him.

Today, however, the words of his father, Mathias Sartor, were loud and clear: *Do not wear down your mother.*

But it was spring! And he was her Pierre. Fortunately, there were others to help care for him. His sister Elise, whom family and friends called Liss, was 26 years old and another mother to him. His sister Lena — her formal name was Helene — was 14. And Pierre had brothers: Ferdinand, 19, and Francois, 17. He knew his brothers would jostle each other and the hale and hearty young men who were their companions during the procession.

Pierre never got roughhoused.

But how could his mother stay calm on such a day? The handkerchiefs had to be readied! In Luxembourg, handkerchiefs can be a form of art. While some may resemble napkins, others are linen confections with decorative lace and elegant embroidery. On this day, it seemed every handkerchief in Luxembourg had to be starched. Why? When people lined up in the procession, row upon row, they would join their hands with the crisp white cloths held in between, like the strings of paper dolls his mother cut for his sisters.

Imagine a mother, trying somehow to keep her three boys from using their starched, bleached handkerchiefs to blot the sweat from their foreheads. Dirty and wrinkled handkerchiefs in the procession would blemish a family's reputation. A lot of apron snapping over that! A lot of arm flapping!

So much for *Do not wear down your mother.* Not with such a day ahead. On some level, Pierre knew, his mother could not be slowed, not today.

Descriptions have come down to us that Catherine Sartor

was "thin and wan." Mother and son shared more than love for each other. Each was in fragile health. Pierre loved his mother and knew St. Willibrord did, too. Pierre's anticipation increased: Surely the good saint could restore his mother to health along with him!

Pierre was familiar with the story of *Hans Brinker, or, The Silver Skates*, a novel published shortly before he was born. It took place in the Netherlands and described a brave and good boy who helped his family because his father was sickly. After many adventures, the father recovered, and a kind doctor helped Hans go to medical school. Would Pierre's story be like that of Hans Brinker?

As his family got ready for the procession, Pierre's conviction grew: He was ready for a miracle. When they reached the Abbey of Echternach, he would ask St. Willibrord to heal him and his mother. Pierre was at the stage of life when the faith and trust of a child blend with the reasoning of a young adult.

Pierre and his mother climbed into the horse cart. Neither would be able to make the walk to Echternach. But Pierre could take the reins with authority.

Mathias marched behind the cart, flanked by Ferdinand and Francois; that's how it was done, the family demonstrating their dignity and solidarity for all to see as they made their way to the procession. It was their happy day, a day off from the fields. Liss and Lena could walk or ride, as they wished.

When I was a youngster, I heard my grandfather Pierre describe the early part of this day, filled with such joy and hope.

Horses pulled their cart at a goodly pace. They went by rows of houses that had been standing together for hundreds of years and ventured into the beautiful countryside.

When they reached the town of Echternach, Pierre's family saw people leaning out windows and over flower boxes a story above the street, like birds in the trees. They passed a shop that sold sweets: red caramel pipes, almond paste and sugarplums.

At last, they came to the town square of Echternach, where families filed into rows for the procession, spreading across the cobblestones. Rows of people practiced their dance, like corn a-popping. They hopped randomly, never all up or down together. Musicians clumped throughout, tooting and whistling, but making no melody as of yet.

Pierre looked at his family as they blended into the growing crowd. He was proud of them. His sisters' skirts were of fabric hand-loomed by their mother and the boys wore smocks called *kittels*, which she had monogrammed. Mama was a skilled weaver. The name "Sartor" means "tailor" and Mathias often told Pierre and his siblings to mind their appearance.

Looking around, Pierre could see some people in the crowd wearing clothes that were coarse compared to theirs, while others had outfits of more elegant fabric and design. What people wore reflected the social order of Luxembourg. Pierre's family were prosperous farmers.

With its close connections to France, Germany and Belgium, the Grand Duchy of Luxembourg had roots in European civilization that predated the Roman Empire. By the time of Pierre's youth, the Industrial Revolution was bringing change — railroads, factories and telegraphs. But for Pierre's family, the traditional ways held fast.

Pierre's breaths burned his chest, and he was only able to hop a bit before he felt wetness in his ears. They were draining again. Pierre stopped skipping, Mathias swooped him up and soon Pierre had a view from his papa's shoulders. Pierre wiped his ears with his sleeves. Ears don't hurt as much when draining, a fact he knew well. From this height, Pierre prayed, looking up into the sky, feeling the warm sun and gentle breeze upon his face: *Please, God, fix me. . . .*

This day would mark the end of the innocence of his childhood.

After riding on his father's shoulders, Pierre was shifted to his brothers' care while Mathias shepherded Pierre's mother. But Papa could not carry her as he had his son. Pierre's worries grew. *Would Mama get better?*

Pierre's day did not go well, and his mother's day was worse. During the procession, she moved ever closer to the end of her row. Then she dropped out of sight as the procession streamed on.

Pierre asked his father: *Mama is out of sight. She must be sitting?*

Best she rest, his father said. They would find her after the ceremony. Mathias lifted Pierre back onto his shoulders so he could keep up with their row as it moved ahead.

The abbey loomed closer. Soon the first rows of the hopping pilgrims went up the steps and inside. The next rows followed as more springers crowded close to the church. The music echoed off the stone walls.

Pierre had to slide off his father's shoulders so his row could enter the church and make its way, down and down, to St. Willibrord's tomb in the bowels of the church. The carvings on the white marble tomb, located below the altar in the sanctuary above, threw shadows.

Pierre swallowed to clear his ears. In the reverberating chamber he voiced his plea for health, for himself and his mother, a prayer that only he and the saint could hear. Before he could say *Amen*, the procession behind him surged forward and he lurched, almost falling onto his face while he prayed. Then he was swept with the throng as it flowed back up the steps to the main part of the church. No cure came.

Now on his knees, Pierre recited the prayers of this holy day as the crowd surged around him. Many of the prayers pertained to health, seeking protection from plague and other maladies. But Pierre didn't understand all of what he was saying — his formal study of Latin would come years later. He could recognize, however, the desperate tone of supplication as people sought cures and help.

Along with the chants and intonations of the ritual prayers around him, Pierre again spoke his petition for health, this time directing it to a statue of the Virgin Mary. With a young boy's eye for detail, however, the image of the day that stuck with him for years to come was of the church organist. That fellow jumped about on his bench like a frog, hopping over his rows of keys and pedals.

The immobile statue . . . the frenzied organist . . . the voices rising and falling around him, beseeching with words he could not comprehend . . . none of this brought the boy close to the saint he trusted to help him.

Pierre's faith was strong, but his ears still hurt.

Sooner than Pierre thought, it was time to loop around the church and out the door, back into the street. How his legs wobbled to keep up. By now, Pierre was disappointed, in a mood so foul that he later described it as sinful. The crushing disappointment that Pierre felt from not being cured was one of the few times when his sense of equanimity failed him. He remembered it for the rest of his life.

The Sartors walked to where they had started the procession and, just as Papa said, Mama was waiting at a wall. By her silence Pierre could tell something was wrong. His mother did not receive a miracle of health that day, either. It was a long walk back home.

Months passed from the early summer beauty of Whit Tuesday through the time of harvest and the coming of winter. Cold, dreary days lingered in that nothing-time after the Christmas and New Year holidays. Pierre's ears still hurt, and his mother was not well.

Then came the night of February 27, 1883.

At the time, Pierre could only wonder: *What is happening?*

Events that strike emotions can last a lifetime.

These are Pierre's memories of the night and day that changed his young life.

I heard him describe those memories on one of his Sunday afternoon visits to our home in Mason City, Iowa, and his painful telling of the fear and grief that he felt so long ago made a lasting impression on me.

As Pierre lay in bed, he knew something was different. The house was strangely quiet, although he could hear muffled sounds. Everyone else seemed to know something. The family left Pierre babied, wrapped in his quilt.

Why hasn't Papa come for my bedtime prayer?

Pierre slept fitfully that night. There were hushed voices,

people coming and going. He heard someone open the front door, much too quietly for their normally boisterous household.

His ears throbbed, felt gigantic. Even his nose stung with a strange drifting scent. It seeped through the dark. Whispered prayers, interrupted by a voice — a low baying like in church, but not so loud as at Mass.

Pierre drifted back to sleep.

Next morning, Pierre got up and made his way into the main room of their house. He took in a scene he could never imagine — and one that he never forgot.

His mother was lying quite still, at full length, on a bed. She was dressed in her finest, hands folded as if in prayer.

Candle smoke plugged Pierre's nose. Where was his mother's scent, redolent of soap and flowers and custard? There was no sweet milk this morning.

The village priest, Father Jean Leysen, was in their house; that was an honor. But . . . the big wooden cross was off the wall. It was next to his mother, flat on the table next to her bed.

It belongs on the wall.

Truth to tell, Pierre himself had taken the cross down on occasion. When no one was looking, he opened the slat on the back that worked like a cover and examined the contents. Pierre knew they had to do with a ritual for the ill and dying. *But I always put the cross back where it belongs!*

Now the priest picked up the cross from the table, slid off the back. He pulled out a candle. He lit it and opened a small pot of oil.

Father Jean dipped his finger in oil and traced a cross on Mama's hands, then her forehead and finally her bare feet; all the while, he prayed. Mama never responded.

Then Pierre knew: His mother was dead.

Pierre had the questions of a child: *When had it happened? Did it hurt?*

Catherine's death shaped Pierre's life. Years later, when he was a physician, he would use the phrase "My heart break" when he lost a patient who was someone's mother. And the rituals of Catholic faith would always sustain him, even when those devotions did not result in a miracle.

He was 11 years old, and now he understood why people wished each other good health and closed their letters with hopes for the same. Health was a gift, a blessing, but it could be gone in a moment.

After Catherine's funeral, the family began adjusting to life without the wife and mother who, in many respects, had been the center of the household.

Liss took up many of Catherine's duties, but it was not the same.

One spring day began much like the others. It was midmorning, and Liss was still in her nightcap. She warmed the milk, stirring as it steamed; she likely also darned a sock while she waited.

Pierre had all day, no hurry. He pushed lumps of his porridge to the edge of the plate, left the center — a soupy mess. Perhaps table manners died, too, with his mother. Bored with his food, Pierre took to sweeping the room, but that didn't last long, either.

He wondered why Papa and his brothers hung about the house this day. *They should be busy in the fields.*

Soon, Pierre would know. Papa called his family together around the table. Something had to be resolved about Pierre, he said, and it was time to discuss plans for the whole family.

What was the plan?

Mathias did seem to have a plan, all around!

A phrase has been handed down in my family: "No martyr Sartors" — our surname, *Sartor*, rhyming with *martyr*. It's impossible to say whether this phrase was in use when Pierre was a boy, and the mild humor of the sound-alike words would have been lost in languages other than English. My brother, sisters and I certainly heard this figure of speech from our father, Guido Sartor, when we were growing up.

Its meaning has connotations of *Don't fuss. Stand tall. Carry on.* There is a practical, stoic quality to the phrase, which does seem to have been a family trait for many Sartor relatives across the generations. One can see it in the plans Mathias made for his children.

For 200 years, the Sartors had farmed their own land. The area is composed of rolling countryside, blessed by a mild climate. Beginning in the 1600s, aristocratic families began to offer land for sale to the ordinary people. Generations of Sartors purchased land when it became available, according to their means. The last of the Sartor land had been purchased in 1806.

It was time for Mathias, having lost his wife, to think about the future. He seems to have been determined to do his best for his children according to the wisdom of the time.

Mathias announced that his property would pass to the eldest child. In their family, this was Liss. Even while Catherine Sartor was living, Liss had assumed caretaker duties, which increased after Catherine's death. These abilities would serve her well in managing the inheritance. Lena, the youngest daughter, was expected to marry and start a new branch of the family.

Mathias took a different approach with Ferdinand and Francois. They were younger than Liss and would not inherit the house and land, so what would happen to them? Traditional avenues for young men at the time included going into the military or the clergy. These were honorable callings, but both brothers had already demonstrated skills in business. However, career options in this direction were limited.

"Har ass Har an Max [ass Max]." "Boss is boss and servant is servant." These words come from a letter written in 1948 by one of Pierre's nephews who lived in Luxembourg. He wrote that "the old . . . proverb is all ways [sic] true." The social and economic constraints implied in that statement would have been even more challenging in the late 19th century when Mathias considered options for Ferdinand and Francois in their homeland.

It would be best, Mathias said, for the two brothers to go to America when they were a bit older. After all, Mathias continued, his own brother Nicholas had gone there. It was the land of opportunity, where land and business ventures were readily available. And the brothers could help each other.

Pierre began to realize that Ferdinand and Francois would be exiting his life.

What about me? Pierre must have thought. He was the youngest of all the Sartor children, and in frail health. This day, he wasn't expecting a miracle.

But then his life changed.

In planning for both of his daughters and his two older sons, Mathias focused on tradition and innovation. Now he called upon vision, which opened new horizons: *Pierre will never be strong enough to work on a farm. Many families pick one child to educate. For us, Pierre will be that one.*

The timing was critical, as it would prove to be at other key junctures of Pierre's life. He had already completed elementary school. It was a mark of the Grand Duchy's commitment to education that even small communities had their own school buildings. Boys typically were taught by a male instructor on the main level of a schoolhouse and girls learned from an unmarried female teacher upstairs. This arrangement was not equitable by today's standards, but it was an achievement in the late 19th century, when many girls in rural areas had no access to formal education. Absenteeism was common in rural communities, where children assisted with farm duties. As a farmer, Mathias Sartor was notable for ensuring that his children received a solid education.

Most youth in Berbourg never went beyond the village school. For Pierre, however, Mathias had greater goals: Pierre would attend the *progymnasium*, roughly equivalent to a middle school. It was located in Echternach. And if Pierre did well, Mathias said, he would go to *De Kolléisch* in Luxembourg City, the Grand Duchy's capital and largest city. Luxembourg did not have a university. *De Kolléisch* was a hybrid institution — roughly the equivalent of a high school combined with college-level courses. It would take Pierre to the top level of education available in his homeland, far beyond the traditional aspirations and attainments of his family.

The littlest brother a scholar?

While his family did not come from an elite background, Pierre and boys like him had access to higher-level education, based upon merit. There was no tuition for attending the *progymnasium*; it was a state school, owned by the government and run by the church. But it was a boarding school, and families had to pay for a student's living expenses. That is why Mathias could offer an advanced education to just one of his children.

The plan that Mathias set forth presented daunting odds. Admission was highly competitive, becoming even more so as students sought higher levels. Pierre had to test at the top of the boys his age to get into the *progymnasium*. Coming from a small village, he would be competing against boys who had more academic advantages — and Pierre was behind in what schooling he had received, due to poor health. Looking ahead, only the best students from the *progymnasium* were admitted to *De Kolléisch*. Once enrolled there, Pierre would face a rigorous program, lasting six years. Pierre would be 21 by the time he finished — a decade into the future — living away from home all the while.

And what would Pierre do with that fine learning? Mathias probably did not address this issue in announcing his plan. He knew that social norms in Luxembourg would limit Pierre's professional opportunities. But with the faith that was a hallmark of his family, Mathias likely trusted that, in time, the right path would open for his youngest son. Pierre didn't even know what he wanted to be, not yet. For a lad from Berbourg, the prospect of living as a boarding student and later going to the capital city may have seemed overwhelming — along with the knowledge that at some point, his two older brothers would depart for America.

There was more.

It was clear, Mathias said, that Pierre's chronic earache had to be treated. Before Pierre could go to school, he would have to see a doctor — a specialist — in Esch-sur-Alzette, the second largest city in Luxembourg, about 30 miles away.

This was no office visit or consultation. Under his doctor's care, Pierre would live there while he received treatment. Mathias did not say how long this would take, and it's likely he did not know. But he announced that Ferdinand would go with Pierre for the duration. They would stay in a boarding-house and not return until Pierre was cured. *You will not come home until well*, Mathias said.

Mathias had already arranged a room for the boys. Their meals could be in the room if Pierre was ill and in the dining room when he felt up to it.

Their father had spoken.

Gott in Himmel! God in Heaven!

The plan was set, right in that moment.

Now Mathias reached up to a cupboard and brought down his lockbox. For many families, a lockbox served as a home equivalent of a safety-deposit box at the bank. It contained his children's birth certificates and official papers of all kinds. As an adult, Pierre would have a lockbox of his own, which he passed to his son Guido, and which eventually came to me.

Church records were in the box that Mathias held, which led to another discussion about Pierre. He might not be back home by the time boys his age received First Communion. Mathias declared that Pierre would make his First Communion in a few weeks — an expression of confidence that Pierre was ready for such an important religious milestone ahead of his peers. It took place on May 9, 1883, during the spring after his mother's death.

For 11-year-old Pierre, it must have been hard to take in all he heard that day. But he was optimistic, given a chance. He always would be. And this time there would be no going back. That was clear.

Pierre's home in Berbourg, Luxembourg, was a row-house structure that combined a residence, barn and other facilities.

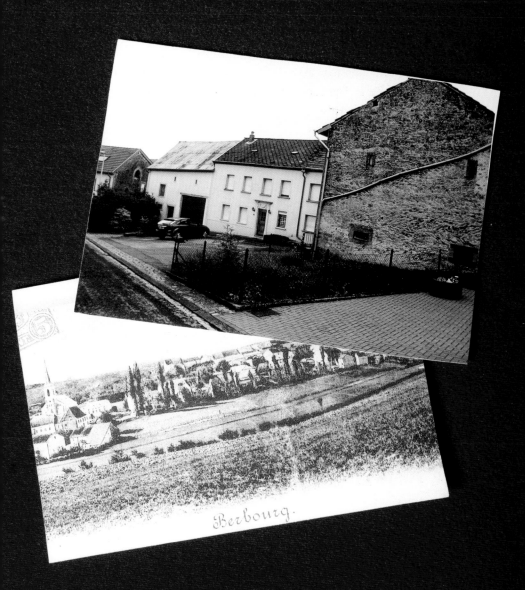

Berbourg.

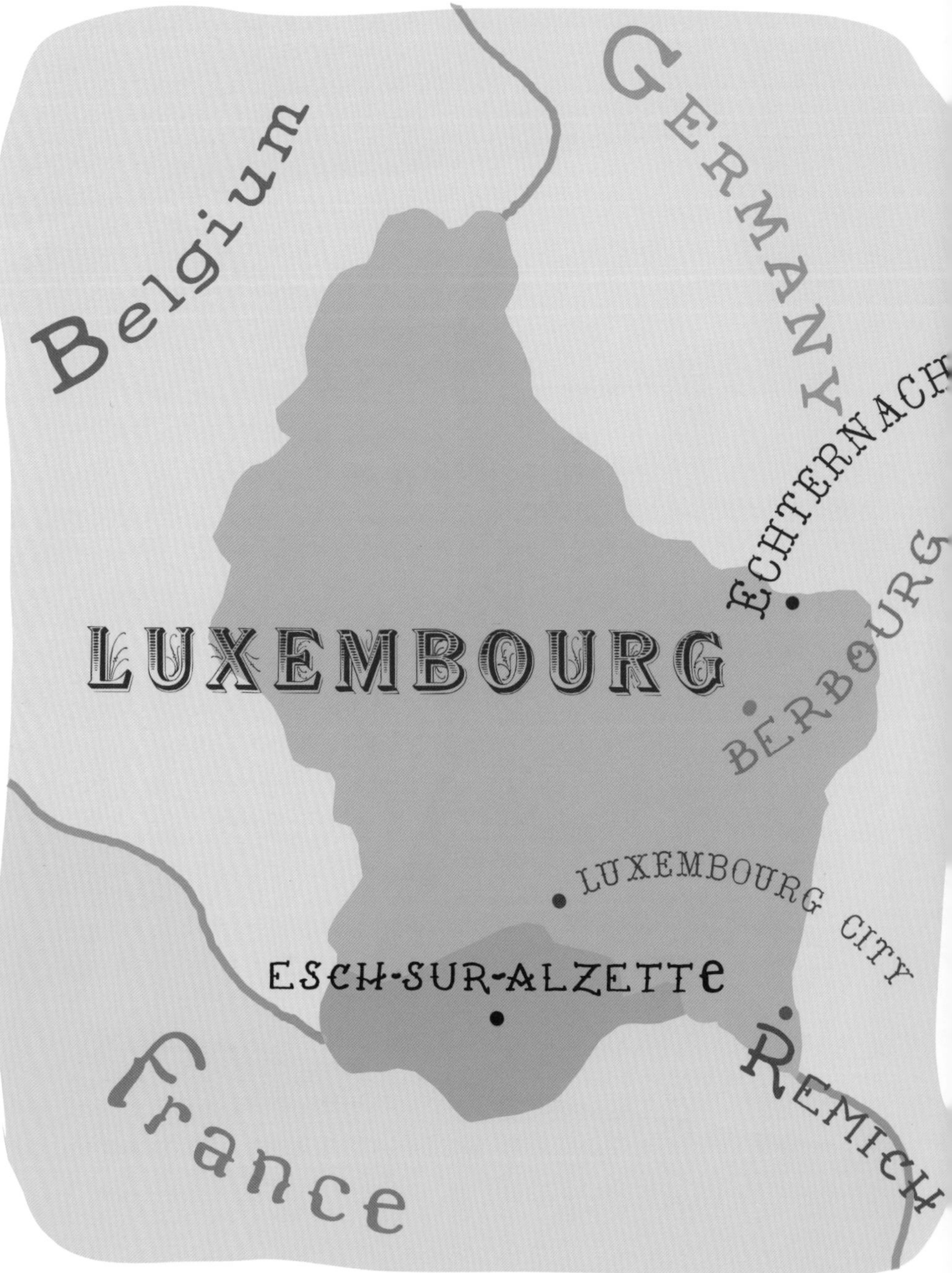
Belgium
Germany
France
LUXEMBOURG
ECHTERNACH
BERBOURG
LUXEMBOURG CITY
ESCH-SUR-ALZETTE
REMICH

Healing, Learning and Leaving

Luxembourg
1883-1893

PIERRE WAS A BOY OF THE COUNTRY, heading out from home.

Liss sorted fruits and vegetables and baked goods, some dried meats. She made trip after trip up the ladder to their loft to pick the best from their harvest.

Ferdinand and Pierre loaded the cart, climbed aboard and began their journey. Mathias walked alongside them. He lit his pipe for the walk ahead.

Other people were out and about. Father and sons may have seen sleighs with runners greased to slide over the road, dogs pulling carts — all manner of vehicles, many of them loaded with stone jars and shiny brass kettles. When a milk cart rattled past, it was best to stay out of the way!

On this journey through the countryside, Pierre thought he was going to a castle in the sky, an easy assumption because

Nestled between Germany, France and Belgium, Luxembourg has a strong, independent spirit. Its national motto is translated as "We want to remain what we are."

Luxembourg has castles spanning several centuries that are acclaimed for architectural beauty and rich cultural heritage. A classic book about the region is aptly entitled *The Land of Haunted Castles*.

In Pierre's mind, it was natural that his doctor's office would be in a castle.

Pierre enjoyed the trip, but sweat dripped down his back, that awful feeling when one is not well. His impressions upon arrival in Esch-sur-Alzette are not recorded. Mathias bid them farewell along with, no doubt, some final instructions. Ferdinand and Pierre settled into their room in the boardinghouse.

Next morning, Pierre nearly fell out of bed! He was used to being in the middle, three brothers in one bed. It was early and Ferdinand tucked him back in. Ferdinand said he would take a walk, find the best route to the doctor's office. Ferdinand embraced the role of caretaker. He also realized that living away from home for the first time would be a great adventure.

Pierre had his own excitement that day, without leaving the room. As he described it years later, he noticed a magazine on a little table. Curious, Pierre opened the publication. His family received no magazines at home, so he was not prepared for the tone and appearance of one story.

The picture on the page was of a man's face. It was not only toothless but the nose was — burned away! Pierre became absorbed and read the story. It described Charles II, King of Navarre, a region in Spain, who had lived in the 1300s. He was known as Charles the Bad for his wicked life. When Charles became ill, his doctor wrapped him in cloth that was soaked in brandy. A servant held a candle too close to the king, causing the cloth to catch fire, leading to a terrible death. At least, that was the tradition.

For a young boy contemplating treatment by a doctor he had yet to meet, the story made a vivid impression.

Ferdinand returned to their room; he had located the doctor's office. Soon, the brothers were on their way to the doctor. They saw tall buildings and the air was thick with coal smoke from chimneys that seemed to fill the sky. A city was compact with hard surfaces, so different from the soft, lush countryside they knew.

When they arrived at the doctor's office, they waited in an outer vestibule. Time slowed, but Pierre's heart raced. For the second time, he had a jarring experience with a magazine.

A medical journal was on the table beside him. Pierre thumbed through it and was appalled to see technical illustrations of patients undergoing treatments that would look frightening to a child. Some illustrations showed a patient being forcibly held down during painful operations or other procedures.

Pierre later said he wished he had not seen such a magazine that day. Would any of those things happen to him?

Ferdinand took the journal, put it away and directed Pierre to a frame on the wall. In contrast to the lurid images in the medical publication, the frame contained the words of the Physician's Prayer, which would comfort Pierre as a child and guide his career as an adult. There are multiple versions of the Physician's Prayer, and while the words vary, the intention and spirit are consistent. At some point during the months he visited the doctor's office in Esch-sur-Alzette, Pierre copied the Physician's Prayer. Here is the version he later used as his personal and professional guide:

> *Dear Lord,*
> *Thou Great Physician,*
> *I kneel before Thee.*
> *Since every good and perfect gift must come from Thee:*
> *Give skill to my hand, clear vision to my mind,*
> *Kindness and sympathy to my heart.*
> *Give me singleness of purpose,*
> *Strength to lift at least a part*
>   *of the burden of my suffering fellowmen,*
> *And a true realization of the privilege that is mine.*
> *Take from my heart all guile and worldliness*
> *That with the simplest faith of a child I may rely on Thee.*
> *Amen.*

Eventually, Pierre was called into the doctor's office. He sat in a chair, and his feet did not touch the floor.

The doctor asked questions. He started gently, conversation-ally: *How are you?* An optimist despite his frail health, Pierre gave his typical reply when anyone asked about his health: *I am good*.

More questions, probing to the nature of Pierre's problem.

A nurse took notes. She and the doctor conversed in French, using medical terminology that Pierre could not follow.

Next question: *Pressure? Were his ears full?* Little by little, Pierre's answers spelled out his condition for the doctor and nurse. The questions got harder.

How long since you could hear well? Pierre could not recall a time when he did not have an earache or a cold, his breathing coming in rasps. Ferdinand backed him up.

The doctor hoisted Pierre onto a table. He poked soft fuzz — and cold metal — into each ear.

After more than a century, one cannot diagnose Pierre's ail-ment with certainty. But it seems likely that he had a condition known as chronic serous otitis media, which involves thick flu-id behind the eardrum and is nicknamed "glue ear." It can sig-nificantly impair hearing. Chronic serous otitis media is com-mon in children who have frequent colds, ear infections, enlarged adenoids and poorly functioning eustachian tubes, which open with swallowing to allow air to enter the space behind the eardrum.

The doctor may have performed a procedure known as myr-ingotomy, which creates an incision in the eardrums, allowing fluid to drain. Although the first myringotomy took place in 1649, the procedure did not achieve widespread effectiveness until the latter half of the 19th century. A professor at the Uni-versity of Halle in Germany published information about the procedure in 1868 and the world's first clinic devoted to ear conditions opened in Vienna in 1873.

The timing and location of Pierre's treatment is significant. Luxembourg, with its proximity to great centers of learning in Western Europe, provided his doctor with access to new, ad-vanced medical knowledge. It's also important to credit Pierre's father with the foresight and determination to seek out a specialist to help his son.

One can discern echoes of this experience in Pierre's future collaboration with specialists, particularly his colleagues at Mayo Clinic. As a community-based practitioner in rural Iowa, Pierre referred patients for specialty care at Mayo, as well as to other hospitals in the region. He incorporated advanced knowledge into his own practice. Pierre's son, my father, Dr. Guido Sartor, did the same.

As he described this meeting in later years, Pierre could not recall the doctor's exact words. But he never forgot the doctor's soft voice — it soothed. The doctor didn't hug Pierre. What he did, however, was priceless. The doctor told the truth and provided comfort.

The doctor was a caregiver.

The doctor said he would observe Pierre carefully to chart his progress. This reminded Pierre of what his father had said. Mathias made it clear that Pierre was not to come home until he was better, however long that took.

The doctor's instructions were simple: Back at the boarding-house, Pierre was to put warm cloths to both ears, allowing them to drain. Pierre was to keep water out of his ears and get plenty of rest.

This became Pierre's daily regimen. In the days and months that followed, Pierre lay on his bed: first on one side, allowing his ear to drain, then switching to the other side, rarely sitting upright. It was tedious but tolerable. With difficulty, Pierre overcame one temptation. The boardinghouse had a large bathtub, great for splashing, but Pierre followed the doctor's admonition to keep water out of his ears.

What Pierre later described of his recovery from the debilitating earache was based upon his senses and emotions as a boy struggling to recover his health. For six months, all Pierre did was wait for his ears to stop draining and make periodic visits to the doctor.

Each morning, Ferdinand rinsed out Pierre's pillowcase and hung it on the open window shutter to dry. Pierre began to recognize the voices below, though they never spoke to him.

Ferdinand went for walks every day. He returned with accounts of people he had seen — girls, hoodlums, the many characters that filled the town. He was a good storyteller.

The time got long, the novelty old. Pierre grumbled more and more. He picked at Ferdinand. Pierre's only contact with the world was from a window. Why did this doctor have to be in such a big town? Couldn't he have an office in a pretty place like home where the forests grew, where animals lived? Where the air was clear, not smoky?

Pierre's comfort was prayer, especially the Physician's Prayer. His favorite verses:

> *Take from my heart all guile and worldliness*
> *That with the simplest faith of a child I may rely on Thee.*

Pierre returned to the doctor's office periodically. With boyish interest, he surveyed the medical and surgical tools that lined the shelves. They were made of metal and gleamed in the light. Displayed row upon row, they looked like so many boars' teeth. Some of the tools reminded Pierre of the needles on a hedgehog.

He was sitting in the doctor's office one day, letting his imagination roam, when the doctor arrived and began what became their most significant conversation yet.

The doctor examined Pierre. He spoke in his matter-of-fact way, but his words riveted Pierre's attention. *Break the eardrums. . . .*

The doctor was so calm. He could have been saying, *Let's go for a walk.*

Who knew, I have drums in my ears! thought Pierre. Nothing in the doctor's office or the medical journal he had seen gave Pierre any idea that there were drums inside his head. It was difficult to imagine.

But the doctor was going to break them? How would he do that?

No purging, begged Pierre. To purge was to have the patient drink something so vile that it induced vomiting that would rid the body of toxins. To his relief, the doctor said he did not believe in purging.

Sweating? Again, the doctor reassured Pierre. He would not use that method.

What about blistering? With this method, a doctor would coat a patient's skin with a plaster that raised a fluid-filled bubble, which the doctor then burst to drain out poisons. No, the doctor said, he would not do that.

The methods that Pierre feared had fallen out of widespread medical use during the previous generation. It is likely that with a boy's sense of horrid fascination, Pierre had heard stories from older adults who described purging, sweating and blistering and then applied those experiences to his own situation. Rather than dismiss Pierre's anxiety out of hand or take umbrage at the suggestion that he might use outmoded treatments, the doctor made a special effort to reassure Pierre.

The kindness that Pierre received in this time of need had a formative impact upon his future life in medicine. A patient who knew Pierre more than 60 years later recalled:

> *We always . . . looked upon Doctor Sartor as a very kind doctor. Many a time he told me how each time he experienced a feeling of reluctance within himself before administering any medicine by needle to a child, because of the possible pain.*

Pierre must have been relieved when his physician ruled out harsh methods, but he still did not know what type of treatment his doctor would use. But he trusted the doctor.

Soon? Pierre asked.

Soon, the doctor assured him. He sent Pierre back to the boardinghouse to rest.

In the days that followed, twilight arrived earlier. The air was crisp. Poinsettias lined the windows of their boardinghouse. Christmas was coming. Pierre said his father's prayer every night.

Schéi Chrëschtdeeg! Merry Christmas! came the voices from below his window.

Oh, to have one of his mother's *boxemännchen*, the little pastry men she made. It was his first Christmas without her, and his thoughts were a mixture of sweet memories and sadness, coupled with anxiety about what his doctor would do.

Pierre did have a memorable Yuletide meal, but it was not at all what he expected.

Since arriving in Esch-sur-Alzette, Pierre and Ferdinand had always seen the doctor in his office. One day, however, the doctor came to their room in the boardinghouse. He sat next to Pierre. Ferdinand and the housekeeper hovered nearby. Ferdinand said that today he and Pierre would not go downstairs for the main meal. Around noon, food was brought to the room.

What a feast! There was Pierre's favorite, *ham am hee*, a Luxembourg classic. "Hee" is hay, wrapped about the ham while it cooks. Pierre even got *träipen*, a black pudding made of sausages, pig's organs and vegetables. And *bouneschlupp*, a soup made of green beans. It was the food he loved, and it reminded him of home.

He had seconds of everything, all the while drinking fine wine from the Moselle Valley, the region in northeastern France, southwestern Germany and eastern Luxembourg whose vineyards are famous throughout the world. We don't know if this was Pierre's first taste of wine — possibly not, since he was approaching adolescence in a culture that prized winemaking. But there was something special — unusual — about this meal.

Again and again, the doctor filled Pierre's glass. Its sparkling crystal facets reflected the winter sun like a kaleidoscope. Pierre was surprised to be treated in such a grown-up way; he was the center of the party. They listened to whatever he said and laughed at all his jokes. And there his memory ends.

The wine acted as a general anesthetic for the surgical procedure that followed. It seems likely that the doctor performed another myringotomy, perhaps removing a section of the eardrum, as one school of thought at the time advocated. There is no evidence that the doctor inserted a grommet to facilitate drainage — another approach used at the time, which was revived as a widespread practice known as "tubes in the ears" in the mid-20th century.

We do know Pierre made a successful recovery, which enabled him to pursue rigorous higher education and a demanding professional career. As an adult, neither Pierre nor the people around him said he had difficulty hearing. Decades after the procedure, when Pierre attempted to enlist in the military during World War I, he was rejected due to his age, not because of any hearing impairment.

In the hours immediately following the procedure, Pierre awoke with a hangover and residual pain from the operation. His feet and hands felt as large as the room, fragile as a balloon — no, make that heavy as sandstone.

Although his recovery seemed slow and on some days he was hot with fever, Pierre began to notice the changes that were taking place. At first, his pillows were a mess, streaked red and yellow, and his ears still throbbed. With time, however, the pillows were clean, and he became aware of the sounds around him.

When his room seemed too confining, Pierre used his imagination to explore . . . in his mind's eye, he was climbing over a stone fence . . . walking to the village square . . . racing over cobblestones . . . chasing his father and Liss. He flew through the clouds and landed at the cemetery by his church. His mother was waiting at the cross over her grave. She opened her arms and became transformed into tiny sparkles. Pierre found this reverie to be comforting. His mother was not gone. She was with him, following along with him. It was Love.

One day, Ferdinand stood at the door to their room and asked: *Go for a walk?* Pierre heard every word! As time passed, his hearing got progressively better.

Trains rumbled by their boardinghouse and now Pierre could hear the whistle clearly. It was so shrill he had to cover his ears. The brothers sang songs to fill the time. Pierre could hear himself and Ferdinand. After barely perceiving muffled sounds for as long as he could remember, Pierre now discovered his brother had a loud voice!

Able to hear more clearly, Pierre realized how much he had relied on lip reading over the years. Now he was through with the frustration he had known all his life, pounding his head on the pillow, trying to make his ears work. And he would never forget the day he heard footsteps!

During his recovery, the gratitude that Pierre felt toward his doctor took on an aura he associated with his mother and with his religious faith. He had received his miracle after all. His mother's love sustained him, God made it happen and the physician was God's instrument in helping Pierre feel better.

"Doctor" would come to mean not just a word or professional title to Pierre, but the foundation of his life.

Now it was Lent, marking the passage from late winter to early spring. Pretzel Sunday came — the fourth Sunday in Lent. Both brothers missed the festivities when boys give pretzels to girls in friendship and, in the way of young people, courtship. On the following Sunday, girls reciprocate by giving painted Easter eggs to boys. Pierre must have wondered, *When can I go home?*

There came a night when Ferdinand spoke in a whisper. It was a test. Pierre heard clearly and answered promptly. Both brothers knew: It was time to see the doctor.

What a different meeting from their first appointment in the doctor's office. The doctor clapped his hands. Pierre jumped. Pierre showed him his handkerchief, and it was clean.

Pierre had been an exemplary patient and the doctor had given the best of his professional service. Now it was time for Pierre and Ferdinand to return home. The brothers had been gone almost a year, which translated into one month for each year of Pierre's life.

The doctor and Pierre said goodbye to each other and wished each other luck. Suddenly, Pierre didn't want to leave.

Then just as suddenly, a thought came to the lad that was so clear and so right it seemed part of his soul.

Pierre Sartor, several months shy of his 12th birthday, decided at that moment that his calling was to be a physician.

The brothers laughed, smiled and cheered as they traversed the countryside, heading home. The trees were as they had left them a year ago in springtime — like upended brooms trimmed with nubs of green. An ox pulled a cart of manure at the edge of a field.

Oh! The ripe, warm fragrance! Not at all like the exhaust of city industry, or the cold essence of steel. Pierre was going back to life and growth, his land.

Even the day played along. The sun pushed the clouds, lighting the fluffy tails, and that brushed his mood. Spring in Luxembourg is exquisite.

Ferdinand promised much on the ride home. Someday, he said, they would skate past beautiful homes, past castles. Pierre would finish his education, and then he would have money.

Ferdinand was already developing a good head for business. He had lived a year in a city, managing the money their father was able to send and caring for Pierre through illness and recovery. Back home in Berbourg, their brother Francois had spent the year honing his skills at bartering and other aspects of business.

But try as he might, Pierre, the youngest brother, was not of that material mind. Pierre was fascinated with his doctor and the way he cared for patients.

For now, though, uppermost in Pierre's mind was seeing his little town again, the humps and hills, his home and family. The hours pounded by in that cart.

And then their family was in sight! The boys jumped off the cart, balancing their bundles on their shoulders and backs.

How Francois had grown! His ankles showed beneath his britches! And Lena's dress had a new shape.

There was big sister Liss, standing alongside Mathias; they looked just the same as before. And Pierre would remember the sensation as, one by one, the family had to touch his ears. They tickled him like he was a puppy!

Liss made the family's favorite meal, just like Mama. Pierre presented gifts to each member of the family. A toy wooden ladder for Lena, with a mouse that flipped this way and that, top to bottom; he'd carved it from twigs. A soap carving of a flower for Liss, after his knife grew dull. He gave the knife to Francois. And a bib for Mathias that Pierre had made from a surgical napkin left in his room.

After the feast, it was time for business. Mathias took off his new bib and folded it into a square, a sign they should quiet down. *Do not forget*, he said, *Pierre is to go to school.*

First things first. Pierre was behind in his education. He would be tutored at home for a year to catch up before taking the entrance examination for the *progymnasium.*

Pierre had received one miracle, which brought him restored hearing. To advance in the world of education, he would need a different kind of miracle.

Pierre learned quickly over the year and enjoyed being home with his family. On one wall, Liss displayed a frame with his First Communion certificate, scrolled in gold. It would hang in each of his homes throughout his life.

When the time came for Pierre to be tested, the results were all that he and his family could have wished. Pierre had one of the best scores among the 100 or so boys who took the admission test. He embarked on the journey of formal education.

That journey took him away from Berbourg to the town of Echternach.

When Pierre arrived on his first day at the *progymnasium*, he must have caught his breath. This school was larger than any place he had studied before, elegant and filled with arches. Inside, the walls had engravings. Even the stairways had chandeliers.

A well-tended courtyard was enclosed within the four sides of the building. The courtyard was edged with a path. Boys walked along the path like little priests, holding and reading from textbooks as they paced. But the sky above was familiar and reassuring, blue with puffy white clouds.

In the dormitory, Pierre slept in a room with 16 cots. A schedule on the wall showed days and hours in rows of squares. Every hour was occupied. Pierre would not be alone for a long time.

Pierre made friends and, as children on the cusp of adolescence do, they discussed their future. A boy named Peter Trierweiler wanted to become a priest and go to America. Mathias

Huss wanted to be a lawyer, also in the United States. Pierre wanted to be a doctor, but he didn't tell everyone just yet.

What he did know was that Papa said if he completed his education, he would have the accoutrements of a professional man: a dignified coat to wear and a desk with an inkstand for writing. Pierre knew he had to get more than passing grades. He had to perform not only at his personal best; he had to achieve top grades among his peers to qualify for the highest-level school, in Luxembourg City.

The academic program was demanding. Between class and study, he would be in one large room from 7:30 a.m. to 9:00 p.m., seven days a week. Even Sundays had six hours of study! Attendance at Mass was a daily requirement. Students were allowed two group outings per week, under supervision. They could go to town one hour each week, also with supervision.

Some boys teased Pierre because he wore a smock, typical attire for a farmer's son. Such humor could be cruel if the boys mocked his social standing, but some of the banter could be good-natured as well. Pierre seems to have taken it in stride, a quality he demonstrated in other challenges throughout his life.

Decades later, Peter Trierweiler, by then a Catholic priest in the Diocese of La Crosse, Wisconsin, wrote to Pierre:

> *I perfectly recollect your name . . . and distinctly re-member your appearance and dress as a student, and I vividly recall you in many scenes of fun and frolic of our school days.*

Pierre's humor was a lifelong gift that served him well, and his independent streak comes out in a further recollection from Father Trierweiler as he described a faculty member:

> *. . . whom you horrified one day by the statement that you were a habitual reader of* le Radical. *In a composition of yours you had used certain modernistic expressions & he asked you where you had gotten those words & your answer was: from* le Radical *and he threatened to denounce you to the professor of religion.*

71

In between his high spirits and exploration of new ideas, Pierre was also a dedicated student, and the hard work paid off. Records that have survived in our family collection show that in 1886, Pierre was first in his class. He earned 1,281 points out of a possible 1,536 — almost 30 points ahead of the boy in second place and 34 and 35 points ahead of the students who were ranked third and fourth in the class.

Later in life, Pierre did not write or talk much about his academic achievements or of the graduation ceremony and any celebration that took place.

We know that Mathias saved the ornate graduation program in his lockbox. It was Pierre's first major academic accomplishment and paved his way to the next level of his education, the Athénée Royal Grand-Ducal in Luxembourg City. Established by the Jesuits in 1603, it is the oldest school in Luxembourg that is still in existence. It has gone by several names throughout its history and today is known as the Athénée de Luxembourg or *De Kolléisch*.

In his interviews and writings years later, Pierre did not reminisce much about this phase of his life. The academic work must have been consuming. The school had stringent discipline and a strict schedule. It was a time of transition and tumult in education as the political and religious leadership of Luxembourg wrestled with how best to adapt education to the needs of an agricultural society that was becoming more commercial and industrial. Pierre's attendance coincided with increased focus on science in the curriculum, which helped prepare him for the medical profession.

While Pierre was in Luxembourg City, changes were taking place for his family in Berbourg.

Fulfilling their father's plan, Pierre's brothers left for America. Francois, the middle brother, went first, in 1890, followed

Although he grew up in a rural community, Pierre earned admission to elite schools in Luxembourg. His name is listed first on the honor roll that is placed over the ornate graduation program.

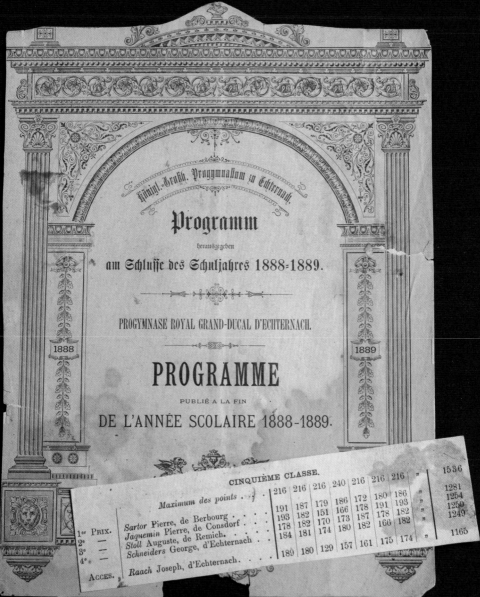

Königl. Großh. Progymnasium zu Echternach.

Programm

herausgegeben

am Schlusse des Schuljahres 1888-1889.

PROGYMNASE ROYAL GRAND-DUCAL D'ECHTERNACH.

PROGRAMME

PUBLIÉ A LA FIN

DE L'ANNÉE SCOLAIRE 1888-1889.

1888

1889

CINQUIÈME CLASSE.

Maximum des points	216	216	216	240	216	216	216	"	1536
										1281
1er PRIX. Sartor Pierre, de Berbourg	191	187	179	186	172	180	186	"	1254
2e — Jaquemin Pierre, de Consdorf	193	182	151	166	178	191	193	"	1250
3e — Stoll Auguste, de Remich	178	182	170	173	187	178	182	"	1249
4e — Schneiders George, d'Echternach	184	181	174	180	182	166	182	"	
ACCES. Raach Joseph, d'Echternach	189	180	129	157	161	175	174	"	1165

by the oldest brother, Ferdinand, the next year. Also while Pierre was away in school, Liss married a farmer named Joseph Rischette. Papa and the younger sister, Lena, were the only ones who still lived in Pierre's family home.

Some days Pierre was homesick, with a sense of urban solitude. He had been far from his family for many years. Sometimes he felt he had only the city itself to be his friend.

Perhaps Pierre's main consolation was the Cathédrale Notre-Dame de Luxembourg, located next door to his school, with its statue of the Comforter of the Afflicted. Dating back to the early 1600s, the church had provided comfort in times of war, plague and famine.

Pierre loved the church, but he did not want to be a priest.

And he grew tired of urban life. He had already chafed at living in Luxembourg's second-largest city, Esch-sur-Alzette, during the year his ears were treated, followed by his studies in Echternach. Luxembourg City, capital of the Grand Duchy, was even larger, an ancient place, over 1,000 years old, built as an impregnable fortress, crowning unscalable rocks.

As a young adult living on his own, Pierre developed perspectives that shaped his future life and career. Several impulses were at odds with one another and would not be resolved until years had passed and he was living on the American prairie, far from the European capital where he was now.

Pierre was drawn to a professional vocation — medicine — yet he found that living in a city, where most doctors practiced, was unappealing. He craved status but was not driven to make money, and his natural empathy was for the poor. He was adept at science and other academic pursuits, while the Catholic faith was central to his life and the ministry of helping those in need was more important than a display of technical skill.

Looking around him, Pierre could make comparisons. A much larger city, Paris, was just 230 miles to the west. The devastating cholera epidemics of the 1830s were part of the collective memory of people he knew, and the accounts he heard took on sharper focus with his developing interest in medicine. Cholera ravaged the poor because of their crowded living conditions and impure drinking water. Stories lingered of wealthy people who continued their indulgent lifestyle in the midst of suffering, believing their wealth and position conferred safety.

Mass outbreaks of disease would surely come again. It was only a matter of time.

To know Pierre is to understand that he would not be satisfied merely to treat an epidemic. He would want to beat it.

During the final year of his studies, Pierre considered his next steps. America offered opportunity for medical education and a career, just as it had for his brothers in their pursuit of business. During the two years since they left, Ferdinand and Francois had settled near Chicago, married, started families and appeared to be doing well.

Pierre wrote to Ferdinand, asking to join him and Francois in the United States.

Pierre's letter went unanswered.

Home for the Christmas season of 1892, Pierre celebrated with Mathias and Lena, joined by Liss, her husband and their children. It seems likely Pierre would have met the new parish priest in Berbourg, Rev. Nicolas Moes, who had begun his duties the previous May.

Father Moes had ambitious plans to construct a new church in the village. With his devotion to St. Roch, protector of the faithful against plagues and other illnesses, Father Moes would have found common ground with Pierre, a devout Catholic who planned to become a doctor.

Thousands of miles away, another member of the Moes family had recently completed a project that would involve Pierre in the years to come. Maria Catherine Moes was born in Remich, about 20 miles south of Berbourg. She immigrated to the United States and entered religious life. As Mother Alfred Moes, she founded a congregation of Franciscan Sisters and led a construction project of her own to aid the ill and suffering: Saint Marys Hospital in Rochester, Minnesota, which opened in 1889. A place of excellence and innovation, Saint Marys would help Drs. William and Charles Mayo achieve international recognition. Later, as a practicing physician, Pierre

75

would visit Saint Marys Hospital and refer many patients to Mayo Clinic.

In 1892, however, Pierre's efforts to reach America were in question. It had been several months since Pierre had reached out to his brothers in Chicago, but he had received no reply.

One day the following spring, when he was back at school, Pierre rushed through the entry of his dormitory as usual. He stabbed his hand into his mail cubicle, as always. Typically, he found nothing. But on that day, he grasped a tissue-thin envelope, postmarked from America.

Pierre slit the envelope. It was from Ferdinand. He wrote in an old German script, which is quoted in translation:

> *April 8, 1893*
> *Dear Brother:*
>
> *We got your letter informing us you will be here to America to complete your studies. We might have answered you, but our business had no time for it.*
>
> *But our job now is going on very well and we make money, and so I can write.*
>
> *Then on March 20th came a young daughter to us. My wife and child are healthy.*
>
> *But our brother Francois's wife, . . . Barbara, adjusts to death of their baby, just one month ago. . . .*
>
> *We . . . send best greeting. . . .*
> *Ferdinand*

The letter was brief; its terms were guarded. Ferdinand and Francois had managed well since arriving in America, but their newfound prosperity and security were at risk. Pierre's correspondence with his brothers coincided with the Panic of 1893, which the Federal Reserve describes as "one of the most severe financial crises in the history of the United States." It swept the country as thousands of businesses and hundreds of banks from coast to coast, including in Chicago, closed their doors.

Against this background of economic crisis, we see the dynamics of the Sartor family at work, which typified other immigrants in American history. The pattern was that some members, such as Ferdinand and Francois, would go abroad to

seek their fortunes. In time, relatives who remained behind —
Pierre, in this case — would inquire about joining them. Alter-
natively, those who moved to America might extend an invitation to relatives and friends back home. An agreement was
needed that new immigrants, as Pierre hoped to be, would be
accepted by their kinfolk who had relocated to America. Such
acceptance would be immensely helpful as the newcomer got
established and could help smooth difficulties as other Americans looked askance at the large numbers of immigrants who
were coming to the United States.

Planning was a challenge because communication took time.
Letters to and from Europe and America went by ship, which
could take weeks or longer. Transatlantic cables had been
available for more than 30 years but would have been prohibi-
tively expensive for Pierre and his brothers. The first transatlantic telephone call would not take place until 1927.

Two months passed. Then, a second letter arrived from Ferdinand. It was undated but more specific — and more promising. After brief pleasantries, Ferdinand got down to business:

> When you have passed your examination, you can
> write us. You deliver your certificate for coming to
> America. You can go to school here not far away from
> the town. You leave in the morning, come back in the
> evening.
>
> What the school cost I do not yet know. I will see
> after it. Tell . . . Father this is our answer.
>
> Also, you did write that sister Lena would like also
> an offer letter, but she not yet written.
>
> Learn English as best you can for there is no Ger-
> man and no French in the school. Only English is the
> principal language.
>
> Our best greetings. . . .

The offer Pierre held in his hand was most generous and gra-
cious. He could stay with Ferdinand and attend a Chicago-area
medical school. Regarding tuition, Ferdinand wrote that he
"will see after it." The meaning was not clear whether Ferdinand would cover the cost or if he would find information

with the expectation that Pierre would pay all or part of his own way.

But it was a good offer, regardless — indeed, Pierre's best opportunity. He had learned from his fellow students in Luxembourg City: *Do not be hesitant. Life gives its fruit to the bold.* His classmates were the cream of Luxembourg's educational system and were expecting to succeed. He would, also.

With his plans taking shape, Pierre now looked forward to spending the summer with Mathias and Lena. He had not lived with his family since the age of 12. He would visit all his old friends and see Liss, her husband and children. While in Berbourg, Pierre planned to earn money for his passage to America and for living expenses once he arrived, perhaps including his medical school tuition in Chicago.

Events took a dramatic turn as Pierre was preparing to leave Luxembourg City for home. He received a third letter from Ferdinand. It communicated reassuring news, and a sense of urgency:

> *July 16th 1893*
> *Dear Brother!*
>
> *After your letter we inquire for cost of the school. It [the education] will take a time. You must go to school here till about four years. It costs 500 francs [$100.00] for a year. We will pay that for you and you can eat with us.*
>
> *In the morning you take the train for the town and in the evening you come back to sleep. We will pay for your books and they will be here as soon as all is in order. You study what you want, doctor or a professor as you like it.*
>
> *But you must not wait until your [summer] vacation is over because school begins one month earlier. You must, will, come over immediately, at the end of your school time.*
>
> *Eight days before your departure, send us a letter with what ship you travel. So we will meet you here in Chicago. At the railway depot you can take a tick-*

et until High Ridge . . . Tell our greetings to Father and sisters and brother-in-law. If Father wants to come, bring him with, and sister Lena, to the trains, and leave them at Paris.

Greetings from us all brothers and sisters-in-law.

Now Pierre knew. His older brother Ferdinand, who had faithfully cared for him through the yearlong hearing treatment, would now host Pierre at his home in High Ridge, near Chicago. Pierre would stay with Ferdinand and his wife, Margaretha, and their baby daughter, Elizabeth, and take his meals with them. Ferdinand would pay for the tuition and books of Pierre's advanced schooling, a level of education far beyond what Ferdinand himself would ever attain. There were no conditions upon this offer, and Pierre had the freedom to "study what you want" in order to become a "doctor or a professor as you like it."

The offer was almost too good to be true, but once again Pierre faced challenges. He must become proficient in English. His knowledge of French and German, to say nothing of his native Luxembourg dialect, would be of little use in medical school. And the next phase of his education would be another long stretch. But before his expansive future in America began, he now had to hurry. Classes began soon. Instead of enjoying vacation and earning money for a comfortable trip, Pierre had to scramble to make life-altering plans according to whatever budget he could manage on short notice.

By this time, Pierre was accustomed to rising to challenges. He reread the three letters many times, following the accelerated commitment that Ferdinand provided. He shared the letters with his family and kept them in his breast pocket, close to his heart. Ultimately, he put Ferdinand's three letters into his lockbox, where they remain today.

High Ridge den 16 Juli 1893.

Lieber Bruder.

Nach deinem Schreiben haben
wir uns umgefragt nach allem.
Die Schule ist nicht theuer.
Aber es nimmt Zeit, ungefähr
4 Jahre mußt du noch hier in
die Schule gehen, die kostet
5 $ das Jahr. Das sollen
wir für dich bezahlen, bei uns
kannst du essen, nimmst den
Zug morgens hier in die Stadt
und abends kommst du wieder
bei uns schlafen. Mache deine
Sachen also in Ordnung und
komme sobald du alles in
Ordnung hast. Wir lassen dich
studieren für was du willst
Doktor oder Professor, wie es
dir gefällt.

CHAPTER 5

Aboard a Tramp Steamer

The Atlantic Ocean
Late Summer 1893

PIERRE'S JOURNEY TO AMERICA was part of a mass migration from Europe in the late 1800s. Ships crossed the ocean, cutting through a curtain of salty air that stung the eyes of immigrants who strained to see the shoreline of their new home. Pierre was 21 years old. He had completed all the education that was available to him in Luxembourg and was ready for a fresh start in America.

What happened en route stayed with Pierre all his long life, and he described it vividly in the years that followed.

The name of Pierre's ship has been lost to history. It was a clunker, a tramp steamer, a hulk of rust with low sides, built long before Pierre was even born.

He stood on a dock in Paris, waiting to board. The ship's route would follow the River Seine for about 130 miles northwest to the Port of Le Havre, from which Pierre's vessel would

On a hazardous voyage across the Atlantic Ocean, Pierre brought these letters from his brother in Chicago, inviting him to the United States.

81

embark for its transatlantic voyage. A huge crane towered over the ship's deck, moving cargo from the dock, up and over to the ship's deck — dropping some crates, gently depositing others. The wooden crates banged incessantly, blending with the chatter and wails of immigrants preparing to leave their families and homelands, in most cases for the rest of their lives.

Amid the tumult, Pierre said farewell to his family. He kept the last words he heard from Mathias close to his heart: *Please remember us in your prayers. But above all, never forget or give up your Holy Mother the Church.*

Faith and the church were ties that could bind across long miles. To the Sartor family, faith meant they would meet again, in heaven if not on this earth.

Having said *adieu* to Pierre as a boy leaving home to receive treatment for his hearing and again when Pierre was a youth heading off to one boarding school after another, Mathias now relinquished his youngest son for the third and final time as a man going to America.

With final hugs from his father and sisters, Pierre stepped onto the gangplank and walked onto the boat.

Once aboard, he stood at the rail in his familiar stance, arms crimped like wings, head tucked under. He watched the crane lift his trunk, bumping it over the horizon, on its way over the ship's deck, and down below to the cargo hold. All around him, passengers crowded shoulder-to-shoulder.

How many people were aboard this boat, a cargo transport that was not even designed to accommodate passengers? No one knew, including the crew who worked the boat and the owners who cut corners to save on costs. Cargo came first, and then immigrants could purchase tickets until the vessel was overfilled. The more passengers, the more profit.

No passenger list, then, and no screening for contagious diseases that could spread easily in the boat's crowded, unsanitary conditions. That some, perhaps many, immigrants would become ill on such a voyage and that any number could die were accepted facts.

But Pierre had worked hard to find this ship. With medical

school starting soon, he had to leave on short notice with no chance to earn money for the trip. His father and his mother's family had done what they could to help him get ready. Across the ocean, his brothers were offering him a home and an education. The ship's ticket had been his to buy, and it represented what he could afford.

His ship certainly wasn't the RMS *Lucania*. Plans for its maiden voyage were in the news while Pierre was preparing for his trip. One of the largest and most luxurious passenger liners of its time, the *Lucania* would make what sophisticated travelers called "the crossing" in five pleasurable days. Pierre's journey would take much longer, in a soul-searing experience he remembered the rest of his life.

A series of heart-jumping booms announced Pierre's imminent departure. In the ensuing thunder, the coal-fired engines came to life. Crew members laboriously turned levers, such as one sees on the door of a bank vault, to close the hatches and lock the water out.

Pierre knew his trunk was down below in the cargo hold. It was well used, and he'd been fortunate to find it. His trunk was a box-size case, flat on top so it could be stacked in the bowels of the ship.

He thought his trunk made him look respectable, and that was important. It had a new coat of shellac. To make a proper start in America, Pierre packed a Prince Albert suit and a top hat.

Pierre also traveled with a satchel, which he kept nearby. As a man of the world, Pierre now had a lockbox of his own, secure within the satchel, containing the important papers of his life. For this moment, the satchel served an additional purpose: He could stand on it, to make him taller at the ship's rail.

Finally, with a tug, the ship started downstream. He would try to put the next moment behind him, leave it in the past, as he was severed from his family.

Pittchen! his sisters called, their voices reaching him from shore.

He felt their love in that name and knew he might never hear it again in their language, their voices. It was a diminutive name. And he was a small man — in stature, but not ambition.

As the ship moved on, his family dwindled to dots.

And then Pierre had time to think. He would have seemingly endless days to think. *What about my brothers? What are they facing, in America? Francois and his wife, Barbara, have lost their baby, an infant of ten months. . . .*

The shoreline shrank away.

Pierre did not know what was in store. But he had a way of never dwelling upon things beyond his control, so he looked ahead.

To become familiar with his surroundings, Pierre went below deck, where he would lodge in quarters for steerage or third-class passengers. His ears burned from the scream of the engine and the bedlam of people around him.

The first night was wretched. Pierre and more people than he could count were crammed into storage space below the water level, where coal and cargo were kept. He remembered the smells, the closeness and roughness of the people, and the ghostly lighting.

Next day, Pierre made his way to the deck. An elegant steamer like the *Lucania* had decks just for promenading. There, passengers could stroll and socialize, enjoy the view and recline in wooden chairs while attentive stewards who wore jackets of crisp white linen brought them lap robes and served tea.

On the deck of his ship, Pierre had to jostle with other passengers for space amid the tangle of ropes, equipment and cargo. In the summer sun, they elbowed for shade, some with middle-class manners and many with less, but any shade was sparse — a pole here, a fluttering flag up there. Pierre found shelter under a canvas, but even there he felt sweat running through his coat. The smokestacks belched gaseous fumes.

Fortunately, on that first day at sea, Pierre overheard that some passengers had a cabin, which allowed them more comfort at night and access to a nicer part of the deck. *After just one night in steerage and one day in the sun, I was convinced to spend my money — and I had enough — to change my ticket.* The change helped, somewhat, but Pierre suffered in the elements. His fair skin and pale eyes were not made for the sun. Heat and salty air made his throat feel like sandpaper. Day or night, the sea could grow wild with waves tossing. Pierre quickly learned the meaning of the term "gale-force squall."

There were moments of absurdity. Once Pierre sat with a group of passengers on the deck near a shaft that led to an opening below. Without warning, a load of coal rumbled down the shaft to feed the engines that powered the ship. In a moment the crowd was covered with soot.

In quiet times, Pierre could reflect upon his surroundings and his hopes. While the passengers endured rough conditions, Pierre saw well-tended wooden crates stamped to mark their luxurious contents: "Lace," "China," "Fragrance." It reminded him of the life he aspired to in America.

When his thoughts turned to food, Pierre's anticipation was less eager. The main meal was at midday. It could be marinated fish with bread and cider or baked tongue, pickled herring, tripe soup, ox kidneys or Yarmouth bloaters (smoked herring). Mystery meals, the passengers called them. *If only I had packed more food*, Pierre thought, but he'd left in a hurry. The steamer had no evening meal, but tea and evening supper were on offer: stewed figs in pudding, at least for a while, until the fruit ran out.

But Pierre did have one advantage to help pass the time. He spoke several languages, which helped him communicate with many of the other passengers. One man was Russian. Pierre found him to be fascinating. The man claimed to be part of a secret society that plotted to assassinate the Russian tsar, or emperor. This was no idle threat. In 1893, the ruler of Russia was Tsar Alexander III. His father, Alexander II, had been murdered a dozen years earlier when members of a secret organization threw bombs at his carriage. Alexander III's son, Nicholas II, would meet a similar fate in years to come. Nicholas was close in age to Pierre, and by the time Nicholas was assassinated, both men would have families with striking similarities.

Pierre also got to know some members of the ship's crew as they swept, oiled, painted and maintained the creaking vessel.

One day, a member of the crew invited Pierre to come below and meet his mates.

We can imagine the mutual curiosity as they got to know each other: men who shared a rough life on the open sea and small, slight, fair-skinned Pierre, who had spent the past decade immersed in books. Even in such an environment, so different for him, Pierre had natural empathy, much as he did for the urban poor who suffered from epidemics. As he said, later in life: *I like people for what they are rather than for what others think they could or should be.*

When he wasn't with the crew, Pierre spent as much time as possible above deck. There were no organized shipboard activities such as on the grand ocean liners. Long hours on a swaying ship under the sky, with little to fix one's gaze, can have a hallucinatory effect. The flag above him — French — gave Pierre some comfort of familiarity.

It was ironic: Pierre had left a country overfilled with people and was now on a boat with passengers squished together like cattle. How Pierre longed to be an angel of mercy. The ailments about him!

The voyage went on. Aboard ships like the *Lucania*, crew members posted regular updates in the lounge to chart the ship's progress across the ocean. As a pastime, well-to-do passengers made bets about when they would reach port. Aboard Pierre's boat, there was no information for the passengers about their location or schedule, and certainly no elegant lounge where they could socialize.

On the open water, it was difficult to get one's bearings. Pierre felt close to the freedom of America, and yet so far. Surely, the shore would appear in due time.

Then crisis struck.

WHAM. The ship lurched. Passengers tumbled. With a rumble and groan and a final screech, the ship came to a halt. Pokey when it was making progress, the ship felt ominous when it stopped . . . and rocked . . . over a world of dark water that seemed to have no bottom. The chug of the steamer, the belch of smoke, the discordant sounds from below, all went silent.

Pierre looked about him for clues, trying to understand the situation. *Where was the crew?* The jovial hard workers whose jokes and tales he overheard any time they came near? His comrades in political conversations when he visited below?

Something was deadly wrong.

For once in his life, Pierre feared the worst and he was powerless to take action. Passengers didn't even have a place onboard to go for information. Pierre prayed to his homeland's patron saint, Our Lady of Luxembourg, *Consolatrix Afflictorum* — "Comforter of the Afflicted."

The events that followed took place over several days. They are a jumble of vivid impressions that come to us from the informal journal Pierre kept aboard ship and the accounts he shared in family conversations and professional presentations over many years that followed.

The most vivid impression was a burial party at sea.

Through salted eyes, Pierre saw it — a procession, crew members up and out of the hold, slowly walking in single file. They carried a body laid out flat on a board, wrapped in canvas. The men brought it to the rail and slid their cargo into the depths of the water. There was no ceremony about what they did, and no captain to preside over the last rites. That is because the deceased was — the captain himself.

Another vivid memory: A crew member climbed onto a platform and asked all those within earshot: *Does anyone have a compass?*

We don't know if the tramp steamer's compass was broken or inaccurate. But it seems that without the captain and his knowledge and skill, the crew was unable to navigate their way.

Pierre's boat was stopped in midocean with no one in charge and no clear sense of how to reach land.

Over the days that followed, order deteriorated. Friendly to Pierre before the captain died, crew members shunned him afterward. They smelled of whisky and kept to themselves. At night they craned their necks to scan the sky. From what Pierre could tell, they were trying to get their bearings using the stars.

On nights when another ship was in sight, a crewman scrambled up a pole and blinked lights as a signal for help. Even on grand ocean liners like the *Lucania*, it would be several years before wireless telegraphy using Morse code became standard, so this limited form of communication was all that was available on the tramp steamer. The signal lamp blinked like a bug trying to attract a mate, but no other ship responded.

Food service on the ship, such as it was, stopped. Pierre went several days eating nothing more than his dwindling supply of wafers. With the Atlantic Ocean all around, he was parched for fresh water. Wedged next to the railing, he had little to do but remember the delicious food he had enjoyed back home.

Finally, when Pierre had stopped counting days — the boat started up. An old sailor finally remembered there was a spare compass stored away on board. The crew fired the engines and the tramp steamer was once again underway.

At last, a shoreline bobbed close, ever closer. They had reached a small island, Miquelon, off the southern coast of Newfoundland. In Pierre's time and today, Miquelon is part of a group of islands that represent the last remnant of the once-mighty French Empire of North America.

With land so close, Pierre's ship had to wait again. Although they had completed their hazardous trip across the Atlantic Ocean with no captain, they needed a pilot to guide them into the harbor of Miquelon. Local fishermen called the fierce currents nearby "the Mouth of Hell." At last, the local officials boarded and guided Pierre's boat safely through the final stretch to port.

Honking geese provided an escort. Passengers lined the railing, eager to disembark after their difficult journey. A glorious sight met their tired, wind-burned eyes — the island's landscape evoked the French Impressionist master, Pierre-Auguste Renoir. Late-summer flowers on shore flickered gold and red in the glinting light and gentle breeze. The trees looked like black sticks with leaves clustered as bouquets of green. For Pierre, it was a remarkable moment of continuity from the Old World to the New.

Soon, an escort boat shuttled up. Just as at the start of his journey, Pierre's trunk bobbled up from the hold and down a line of parcels, until it stopped on shore. Pierre stepped off the plank and onto solid ground. He turned for one last look at the French tramp steamer, which would continue its journey along the St. Lawrence River to Montreal.

Never again did he want to be so powerless, so close to losing so many lives, with people in crisis all about him. He had faced death on the ocean, which reinforced his sense of new life and purpose in America.

The next day he resumed his journey, heading by railroad to Detroit and then Chicago and keeping his brothers apprised of his schedule by telegram.

Conscious of appearance but clueless about how things were done in the American Midwest, he packed away his coat and changed into his best smock — a loose-fitting blouse worn over trousers — woven by his mother, with his initials embroidered on the hem pocket. He had no idea how odd he must have looked to the people who jostled around him.

Those he met had another reason to stare at Pierre. Fluent in French, German and the dialect of Luxembourg, Pierre had a halting command of English at this point. While he could articulate the names of large, familiar cities like Detroit and Chicago when he sought information to catch the right train, he could not make himself understood when he tried to buy his ticket for the last leg of his journey.

High Ridge, he tried to say to the railroad agent, giving the name of the semirural community near Chicago where his brothers lived.

Hi R-r-r-rich! the man behind the bar of the ticket window repeated. He rolled his "r" like Pierre, finding humor in this earnest young man wearing such an unusual outfit.

One day Pierre would tell the story of how he concluded his journey from Europe to America. With characteristic modesty and good humor, he explained: *I would never know if my luck in getting to High Ridge was because of my good English — or my fine Luxembourger clothes.*

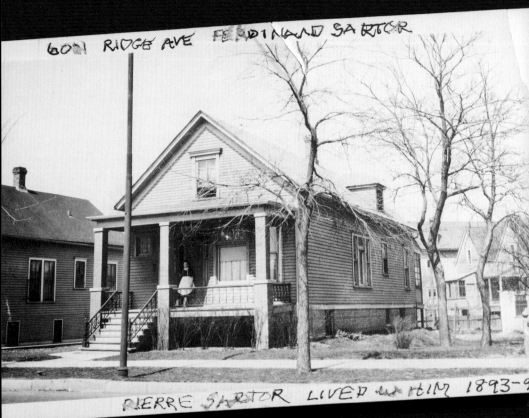

6021 RIDGE AVE FERDINAND SARTOR

PIERRE SARTOR LIVED WITH HIM 1893-9

CHAPTER 6

First Impressions and the World's Fair

Chicago, Illinois
1893-1896

DID THEY CALL OUT TO HIM AS PIERRE, his given name, or Pittchen, his family nickname? Perhaps they hailed him as "Peter," the Americanized version of his name, to welcome him to his new home. However his brothers greeted him as he stepped off the train, Pierre was soon enveloped in hugs and handshakes from Ferdinand and Francois.

After an ocean voyage far more difficult than he could have imagined, and a train trip from eastern Canada to the Midwestern United States, Pierre had reached his destination, High Ridge, a rural enclave north of downtown Chicago. Being met at the train by his brothers gave the strange new place a feeling of home.

In short order, they got to the buggy. Pierre's brothers were eager to bring him up to date. They were partners in a business that built greenhouses for prosperous families in the booming city and its environs. Another part of their business was to sell

From 1893 to 1896, Pierre stayed in this house with the family of his brother Ferdinand while attending medical school in Chicago.

fresh flowers, which were cultivated in greenhouses they rented from Michael Winandy, a fellow immigrant from Luxembourg who had the largest greenhouse business in the area.

Pierre took it all in, but he must have been absorbed by the little cakes that his brothers brought for the trip, in fluted parchment, no less! Pierre was embarrassed to appear so hungry. But at last he could relax; his brothers would keep track of his trunk and satchel.

Excitedly, his brothers sketched out their plans for Pierre, confirming what Pierre had read in their letters earlier that year. While he attended medical school, Pierre would stay with Ferdinand and his wife, Margaretha, and their baby, Elizabeth, at their home in High Ridge, which was home to a colony of immigrants from Luxembourg. Francois and his wife, Barbara, lived nearby. They had recently lost a child and were expecting another.

The homes and lots in High Ridge were so much larger than Pierre had known. His first glimpse of Ferdinand's property was the garden in full bloom on this late-summer day. It was similar to the garden at the Sartor family's home in Luxembourg, but this garden was decorative, for pleasure; it was not intended as a flower crop to be harvested for income. Ferdinand's house reigned over a flight of steps, another surprise for Pierre, since their house in Luxembourg faced directly onto the street.

As the carriage drew up to Ferdinand's house, Margaretha opened the front door. With her words of welcome came an aroma more delightful to Pierre than whatever cologne this elegant lady might have been wearing. Pierre smelled beef stew!

But the rich dinner Margaretha was preparing was not on the menu for Pierre. Simple foods, she said, were the best way to transition from his long trip. With a gentle touch to Pierre's arm, Margaretha explained she would have a meal made just for him when he joined them at dinner, and she would continue doing so for the next few days.

"Invalid cookery" was the term for what she was providing, but the selections Margaretha described — oatmeal, tea, sponge cake, jellies and custards — sounded heavenly to Pierre.

Pierre was used to hospitality in Luxembourg. But this was so much more. Pierre soon realized that Margaretha was a caretaker. She wasn't a doctor like the specialist who had treated his hearing problem, but she was capable and kind, focused on restoring his strength and spirits.

He was fascinated with his sister-in-law in her fashionable dress and crisp apron; her hair was swept up, with wisps escaping across her smooth cheeks. In the future, Pierre would court another young lady in this close-knit neighborhood of immigrants from his homeland: lovely and strong, a capable partner who could adjust to life as it came.

Margaretha took Pierre on a tour of the house. It was the first time Pierre had a room of his own. A curled iron headboard on the bed! Bookshelves. He even had a desk — perfect for his pen and inkstand. Pierre spent an hour cleaning up and dressing for dinner. He never forgot that return to civilization. It reinforced his conviction that cleanliness was the start of good health.

Dinner that night had a dreamlike quality . . . the linen tablecloth, china and silver . . . the spirited conversation as they made plans for the future. The brothers had chosen Bennett Medical College of Eclectic Medicine and Surgery for Pierre because it was nearby and had the endorsement of Francois' physician, Dr. Lentes. Pierre learned that Francois had made a special appeal for him to be admitted. Francois persuaded the officials at Bennett that Pierre's studies in Luxembourg City — six years, with excellent grades — were the equivalent of high school and two years of college. As a result, Pierre was accepted at Bennett before he reached America.

A publication from Bennett Medical College and Hospital that is in our family archive provides information about why Francois was pleased with the selection of Bennett, and why in his letters to Pierre in Luxembourg he urged Pierre to make haste in coming to America:

> *The facilities of this institution for imparting medical and surgical instruction are thorough and complete*

in all the departments, including ample Hospital, Clinical and Laboratory advantages. The annual Term of Lectures commences in September of each year, and continues six months. It is of the greatest importance that all students be present at the beginning of the Session.

Early the next day, Pierre, his brothers and their families walked to St. Henry Church, near Ferdinand's house. Afterward, they strolled through the cemetery. Francois said that someday they would all be buried there: the three Sartor brothers, their wives and children.

Pierre was eager to get established in his new homeland, but that was rushing things a bit!

It would be two weeks before medical school began, giving Pierre time to settle in. He acclimated quickly. Before long, Margaretha stopped preparing invalid meals and Pierre was enjoying the bountiful fare of her table: recipes from Luxembourg with a dash of American cuisine.

There was a special meal on August 23. It was Pierre's 22nd birthday. The cake on Margaretha's platter was traditional, the same that Liss, the older sister in the Sartor family, made back in Luxembourg, with walnuts atop. Gathered around the table in Chicago, they toasted their relatives across the Atlantic. Then they toasted Pierre, newly arrived, with his future before him. Unspoken but deeply felt was the hope that Pierre, the youngest brother and frailest member of the family, would be successful in America. As Pierre acknowledged their good wishes, he felt he had received an entire country for his birthday. It strengthened his resolve to make his family proud. He would succeed — on his own terms.

Pierre's first week in High Ridge flew by, meeting people, getting acclimated. Ferdinand and Francois introduced him to friends and neighbors as their younger brother who was going

Pierre enrolled at Bennett Medical College, which later became part of Loyola University.

94

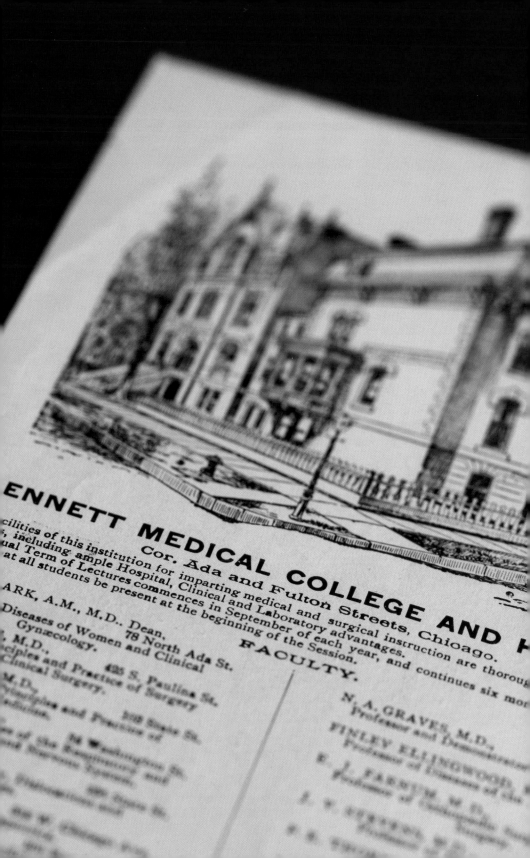

ENNETT MEDICAL COLLEGE AND H

Cor. Ada and Fulton Streets, Chicago.

cilities of this institution for imparting medical and surgical instruction are thorou
s, including ample Hospital, Clinical and Laboratory advantages.
ual Term of Lectures commences in September of each year, and continues six mor
at all students be present at the beginning of the Session.

FACULTY.

ARK, A.M., M.D., Dean. 78 North Ada St.
Diseases of Women and Clinical
Gynæcology.

M.D., 425 S. Paulina St.
ciples and Practice of Surgery
Clinical Surgery.

M.D., 102 State St.
rinciples and Practice of
edicine.

e of the 74 Washington St.
Diseases of

M.D., 305 State St.
W. Chicago and

N. A. GRAVES, M.D.,
Professor and

FINLEY ELLINGWOOD,
Professor of Diseases of

E. J. FARNUM, M.D.,
Professor of

J. V. —

F.

to be a doctor.

As Pierre prepared for medical school, he came to a greater understanding of the environment in which his brothers lived and worked. The Panic of 1893 was a concern. It filled the newspapers. Yet High Ridge was not as affected as some communities because the townspeople were self-sufficient, even raising much of their own food. Also, Ferdinand excelled in business, even in difficult times. During his first two years in America, he had gone from renting a greenhouse to owning one, and he was preparing to buy another. He was an excellent mechanic who could keep the greenhouse operations running smoothly. He was practical and pragmatic, and he made friends easily. Clearly, Ferdinand had built upon the independence and judgment that had enabled him, as an adolescent, to care for Pierre during the year they lived apart from their family for Pierre's treatment.

But not every conversation at the Sartor dinner table revolved around business and medical school. Ferdinand and Francois were full of enthusiasm for the Chicago World's Fair, grandly titled the World's Columbian Exposition, which ran from May 1 to October 30, 1893. It covered nearly 690 acres that featured about 200 temporary buildings in neoclassical and other elegant styles, along with canals and lagoons, and exhibits from 46 countries and cultures. The fair commemorated (one year late) the 400th anniversary of when Christopher Columbus reached the New World in 1492. Pierre, one of the newest arrivals in America, reached Chicago while the fair was in full swing. His brothers said they must go. It was guaranteed to be an inspiration.

Ferdinand and Francois talked in superlatives about the fair, repeating the vivid descriptions of its promoters. Chicago had just earned the nickname "Windy City" — not for its climate, but for the fervor of local dignitaries in wooing the fair's officials to award the exposition to Chicago. The fair was intended to put Chicago on the map — and show the world how, in barely 20 years, it had risen from the ashes of the Great Fire of 1871.

Pierre had the mind of a scientist and a warm sense of humor, so he must have enjoyed bantering with his effusive brothers. We don't know if Pierre had attended the previous World's Fair. The Exposition Universelle was held in Paris at the same time when Pierre was studying in Luxembourg, in 1889. Whether or not he went, Pierre likely knew enough to discuss the comparative features of each fair, particularly their soaring keynote attractions: the Eiffel Tower in Paris and the Ferris wheel in Chicago.

Pierre was eager to see the fair. They chose August 26, the last Saturday of the month. Appearances were important, and Pierre would need a new haircut, one that would serve when he began medical school. It may have been the first time Pierre used the American idiom that became one of his favorite exclamations for the rest of his life: *By golly!*

When the big day arrived, the Sartor brothers swung onto the train that took them from High Ridge into downtown Chicago. Pierre dressed up well, his brothers said. He fit into the clothes that Francois had lent him. The brothers or their wives may have dropped a hint that Pierre should leave the formal top hat and Prince Albert coat he had brought from Luxembourg at home; the derby and business suit belonging to Francois would be perfect this day.

The following would make a great scene in a movie, but it happens to be true: Unbeknownst to Pierre, his future spouse and the love of his life was riding on the same train to the same destination. Mary Magdalene Winandy was 13 years old, nine years younger than Pierre. She was well chaperoned by members of her family, who also lived in High Ridge, as they traveled to the World's Fair.

This cherished moment in the Sartor family lore evokes the classic "Trolley Song" in the MGM movie musical *Meet Me in St. Louis*. That film depicts a fictional group of young people riding a streetcar to another World's Fair, held a decade later in St. Louis. "Clang, clang, clang went the trolley," the character of Esther Smith (Judy Garland) sings as she kindles her affection for the boy next door, John Truett (Tom Drake), while their fellow passengers harmonize:

> With my high-starched collar and my high-top shoes
> And my hair piled high upon my head
> I went to lose a jolly hour on the trolley
> And lost my heart instead
> With his light brown derby and his bright green tie
> He was quite the handsomest of men
> I started to yen so I counted to ten
> Then I counted to ten again.

It would be several years before Pierre and Mary met and fell in love, and no one broke into song while their train made its way to Chicago. But Pierre could not help noticing the easy informality of the people about him. Several women in their late teens and older were unaccompanied by a male escort. Ferdinand explained that in America, women could hold jobs and make their own decisions about where to go and what to do.

When Pierre got off the train with his brothers, he was immersed in the swirl of America's fastest-growing city, chronicled by Donald L. Miller in *City of the Century: The Epic of Chicago and the Making of America*. The fair brought the world's attention to Chicago, barely 60 years after its incorporation and just two decades since the Great Fire. Chicago presented a dizzying array of contrasts: skyscrapers and slums . . . industry and commerce that harnessed the latest technologies . . . ostentatious displays of wealth and strivings for high-toned culture . . . but also corruption, crime and crusades for reform.

It would be 21 years before Carl Sandburg published his poem "Chicago," but Sandburg's description resonates with Pierre's first impression of the "City of the Big Shoulders":

> Come and show me another city with head lifted singing
> so proud to be alive and coarse and strong and cunning.

Pierre's reaction that day, which would be reinforced in the years to come and ultimately inform his decision about where to live and work, was guarded. To a young man from the village of Berbourg, who had considered Luxembourg City large and impersonal, Chicago — "stormy, husky, brawling" in

Sandburg's phrasing — must have been overwhelming.

Despite the new buildings in view, it certainly was dirty. Pierre, always fastidious and now preparing for a medical career, quickly discerned the public health risk from the horses that filled the streets. Their droppings — and their carcasses — fouled the air. Living conditions for humans were not much better. Pierre compared high-rise tenements to "chicken coops," a description he used for the rest of his life, repeated so often that decades and even generations later, his family recalled it.

But if the reality of Chicago was unsettling, Pierre's discovery of a make-believe world fired his imagination. The family says it helped shape the future direction of his life.

It happened by accident.

As the Sartor brothers made their way through the city, they came upon crowds, music, fluttering banners and garish posters that promised a myriad of amazements. They thought it must be the World's Fair. Actually, it was another form of mass entertainment: Buffalo Bill's Wild West and Congress of Rough Riders of the World.

This production was part of a genre that lasted from roughly 1870 to 1920. Wild West shows presented a romantic and sensationalized image of the American West. On this day, the brothers were caught up in the spectacle of daredevil horse riders and other blood-tingling events.

Pierre was mesmerized by Annie Oakley. Petite, feminine and an exceptional sharpshooter, Oakley was a star of the show. She demonstrated athletic prowess and command of her environment in a way that captivated Pierre, who described the experience decades later. She had recently performed for European royalty and as a strong advocate for women's self-defense, Oakley offered to train a women's sharpshooting unit for the U.S. military. A year after the Chicago World's Fair, Thomas Edison recorded her in one of the first motion pictures; her name continued in show business long after her death, particularly with the stage and film productions of *Annie Get Your Gun*, featuring the music of Irving Berlin.

Pierre's first impression of the American West at Buffalo Bill's extravaganza nearly coincided with an utterly different performance on the same topic in the same city. Barely six weeks before, on July 12, 1893, Frederick Jackson Turner, Ph.D., had used the Chicago World's Fair as his platform to read a scholarly paper on "The Significance of the Frontier in American History." Turner's thesis held that the frontier — geographic and conceptual — was key to shaping the American experience. Pierre's future moves westward align with the frontier spirit that Turner described — but Pierre sought opportunities for service rather than conquest.

The brothers eventually left the Wild West show and found their way to their intended destination. They became three of more than 27 million people who visited the World's Fair during its run, taking in marvels such as a moving walkway, a chapel with Tiffany glass and the Ferris wheel. The fair also represented that era's stringent racial segregation, and civil rights leaders such as Frederick Douglass called out the lack of an African American exhibit.

As night fell, the abundant use of electricity — unavailable in most private homes of that time — bathed the classical, ivory-colored buildings in light, which gave the fairgrounds its nickname, "the White City."

As an aspiring physician, Pierre would have been interested in the medical devices on display in the exhibition halls. Other doctors made their way to the World's Fair, including two brothers, William J. and Charles H. Mayo, who took a train from Rochester, Minnesota. Their careers would connect with Pierre's in the years to come. Dr. Will and Dr. Charlie, as they were known to all, were a few years older than Pierre and already establishing a name for themselves at Saint Marys Hospital, which had opened just four years earlier.

The Mayo brothers spent part of their time at the fair on a shopping expedition: "As a gift to Saint Marys Hospital, the Mayos bought a complete set of operating room equipment in glazed enamelware manufactured in Berlin. They brought it from the World's Fair in Chicago."

Pierre did not cross paths with the Mayo brothers at this time. But upon reflection, we can see that this day opened a window to Pierre's future. An impressionable newcomer, he felt hesitant about big-city life, drawn to the American West and stirred by a confident, capable woman.

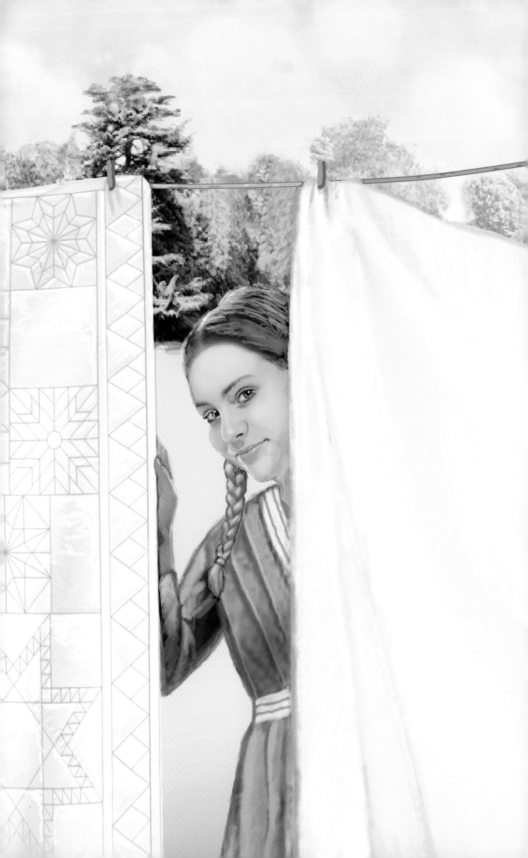

CHAPTER 7

Matters of the Heart: Medical School and Romance

Chicago, Illinois
1893-1898

THE DAY WAS HERE, what Pierre had come to America for — by his reckoning now, what he lived for: his first day at Bennett Medical College of Eclectic Medicine and Surgery. Pierre reached the High Ridge station in time for the early train to Chicago. He stepped aboard with easy assurance — he and Ferdinand had already made a scouting trip to find the right platform for his departure.

Always sensitive to appearance, Pierre radiated confidence as he exited the train and made his way to Bennett. With a freshly pressed suit, he had arrived — not only at medical school but also on the threshold of his future.

Pierre was infused with a sense of purpose. He felt he had been rescued from the malady of his ear problem by the doctor who treated him in Luxembourg and from a life of toil by his father, who decided he would receive an education. Gratitude

At age 15, Mary Winandy was smitten with the handsome medical student who passed by her home. It would be inauspicious to meet him while hanging the laundry, so she gazed at Pierre through wet sheets.

for his own well-being and compassion for the suffering of others inspired his sense that medicine was his calling.

At the same time, Pierre was attuned to the rapid advance of medicine as a science: When he was a child, people turned to folk cures; in 1885, while he was an upper-level student in Luxembourg City, French chemist and microbiologist Louis Pasteur developed a vaccination for rabies "and the era of preventive medicine had begun." During Pierre's time at medical school in Chicago, the German physicist Wilhelm Röntgen would discover the X-ray.

It was a period of transition in medical education.

On one hand, progress: Concepts such as the germ theory were gaining acceptance and moving medicine toward a more scientific basis. Whereas rote memorization had been a traditional means of medical education, the focus was shifting to cultivate medical students as critical thinkers and problem solvers who were actively engaged in lifelong learning. In his personal values and professional career, Pierre represented this new approach.

On the other hand, disarray: Political infighting in 1891 had forced the resignation of the progressive secretary of the Illinois State Board of Health, John Rauch; his successors did not stop the proliferation of poor-quality medical schools in the state. During the 1890s and early 1900s, more than 20 new medical schools opened in Chicago. Some had laudable aims but limited resources, while others were little more than diploma mills. Pierre found himself in a large and growing population of Windy City medical students.

Bennett Medical College of Eclectic Medicine and Surgery had opened in 1868. According to a history of the school, following its destruction in the Great Chicago Fire of 1871, "a large, commodious structure" was constructed at the corner of Ada and Fulton Streets. "To better facilitate the clinical and bedside teaching, a hospital was built directly connected with the college building." A Bennett publication from Pierre's time at the school lists some two dozen faculty members with specialties in a wide range of medical and surgical disciplines as well as related fields such as medical jurisprudence and life insurance examinations.

Under the leadership of Dr. Anson L. Clark, who served as president and dean of Bennett from 1872 to 1905, students had advantages that included attending privileges and access to internships at Cook County Hospital.

At the time of Pierre's enrollment, there were three broadly defined types of medical education. The first consisted of "regular" medical schools, which often were associated with universities. The second type of medical education was "homeopathic." According to this theory, drugs that caused specific reactions in a healthy person should be used to treat the same symptoms in an ill person (*Like cures like*); also, homeopaths believed, the potency of a medication could be strengthened by a series of dilutions.

Bennett fit into the third type of medical education. "Eclectic" schools endeavored to select the most effective treatments from among all therapies that were available. More than a decade after Pierre's graduation and following a critical assessment by Abraham Flexner in his landmark report to the Carnegie Foundation, "Medical Education in the United States and Canada," Bennett and several other medical organizations would affiliate with Loyola University of Chicago. According to a history of the university, "The Loyola University Medical Endowment Fund listed them all and indicated that it was 'happy to claim as her own' all the alumni of these many schools." Known first as Bennett Medical College of Loyola University, the school was renamed Stritch School of Medicine of Loyola University in 1948.

Pierre was one of the first students to enter the building that morning. He took time to adjust to his surroundings.

Looking around, Pierre must have realized he was in for a different type of education. He had attended prestigious schools in Luxembourg that were run by the Catholic Church in a society whose population was virtually 100% of that faith. Bennett was distinctly secular — there were no statues of saints on display, not even the Physician's Prayer, which had been such an inspiration to Pierre as a patient and served as his guide for choosing medicine as a career.

If Pierre noticed pictures on the wall, perhaps he observed women and African Americans in some of the group portraits of previous classes. His own class included several women, something he had not experienced before. Bennett was coeducational from its inception and the student who graduated with highest grades in Pierre's class would be a woman, Mary Elizabeth Bliss, M.D. *The Encyclopedia of Chicago* states: "Like their regular counterparts, Chicago's homeopathic and eclectic schools accepted a small contingent of African American students," but their professional opportunities were increasingly constrained by segregation that would be upheld by the United States Supreme Court in its infamous decision of 1896, Plessy v. Ferguson. That ruling sanctioned the concept of racially "separate but equal" facilities and services until it was overturned more than half a century later.

As the hall filled with students, the voices around Pierre also reflected cultural differences. Pierre had some knowledge of English, but not equivalent to his fluency in French, German and the dialect of his native Luxembourg. The students spoke English with a variety of accents and a strong infusion of slang — code words that Pierre could not crack.

It's possible that he struck up a conversation with a fellow student, John Dill Robertson. A native of Pennsylvania, Robertson worked as a telegraph operator and enrolled at Bennett after moving to Chicago. Even as a young man in medical school, it's likely that Robertson displayed some of the traits that enabled him to blend medicine and politics throughout his career. As president of the American College of Medicine and Surgery, Dr. Robertson would play a key role in the multi-institution merger, which included Bennett, to establish the medical school at Loyola University. A regent of the university wrote of Dr. Robertson, "Loyola University can never repay [him] for his magnanimity in dealing with us."

John Dill Robertson and Pierre Sartor embarked on different paths after graduation, but as physicians, they both confronted the great health crisis of their time. During the 1918 influenza pandemic, Dr. Robertson was City Health Commissioner of Chicago while Dr. Sartor practiced in rural Iowa.

The academic restructuring of Loyola University and the worldwide outbreak of influenza were years in the future when Pierre and John began their medical studies on a September morning in 1893. Pierre's challenge that day was modest compared to the obstacles he faced later, but it was daunting enough at the time. How would he fit in? Could he keep up with the other students, who were fluent in English?

By now the corridor was full. Pierre followed the crowd and settled into the large lecture hall. Rows of seats, arranged on a set of ascending steps, formed a semicircle around the professor below.

Soon the professor spoke. Many of the terms he used were in Latin and German, and the students who responded used similar words as well. Pierre began to relax. The accents were new to him, but the vocabulary was familiar. Pierre realized that his classical and science-infused education in Luxembourg had given him a solid foundation for medical school in America.

Pierre was a diligent young man. He focused as much effort on matters of the heart — romance, in this case, rather than cardiology — as he did on his coursework.

It's a good thing he was so dedicated because Victorian courtship was a labor-intensive, stylized ritual. Pierre's love life was the story of one near miss after another — until he received an assist from a seven-year-old Cupid in the form of his beloved's kid brother.

We don't know exactly when Pierre Sartor and Mary Magdalene Winandy first became aware of each other, but we may date it to the summer of 1895, with Pierre anticipating graduation from medical school the next spring. Although they had been strangers on the trip to the World's Fair, they lived in the same neighborhood in High Ridge and were parishioners of the same church, St. Henry. At some point, their lives entwined.

Pierre forged new paths on his neighborhood walks, just as he would in his career. He took to cutting through the spacious yards, admiring well-tended gardens. Like his brothers, many residents in High Ridge were from Luxembourg and enjoyed horticulture. The Winandy residence, however, stood out. It had one of the largest greenhouses Pierre had ever seen — remarkable, because Pierre had grown up with farmers who raised flowers for a living and both of his brothers were in the greenhouse business.

The owner of this impressive home, Michael Winandy, had one of the most successful greenhouse businesses in the Chicago area. From dinner parties to debutante balls, from hotel lobbies to political conventions, fresh flowers were in demand in the booming city of Chicago. Winandy owned most of the greenhouses in the area. He tilled about eight acres of land, nearly half of which was under glass.

About the time of Pierre's afternoon perambulations, Mary would just happen to appear on the front porch of her home, carefully dressed and coiffed. She would recline in the glider, nonchalantly reading a book or perhaps doing fine needlework as he passed by. In the summer of '95, she was 15. The adolescent girl who rode the train to the World's Fair had become a young lady; Pierre turned 24 in August.

The lad walking about and the young lady on the porch had clearly taken note of each other.

Their yearning courtship recalls how the character of Freddy Eynsford-Hill wooed Eliza Doolittle in stage and screen productions of *My Fair Lady*. Freddy's song, "On the Street Where You Live," takes place in the elegant Mayfair district of London. In the suburbs of Chicago, Pierre, with his smooth cheeks and handlebar mustache, a cape oh-so-casually draped over his shoulders, certainly fit the bill.

Observe each other they might, but there was no conversation as Pierre walked along the street where she lived. In this rarified society, eligible young people must have a proper

As a youngster, Alfred Winandy (below) was the mischievous Cupid who brought his sister Mary (above) and Pierre together.

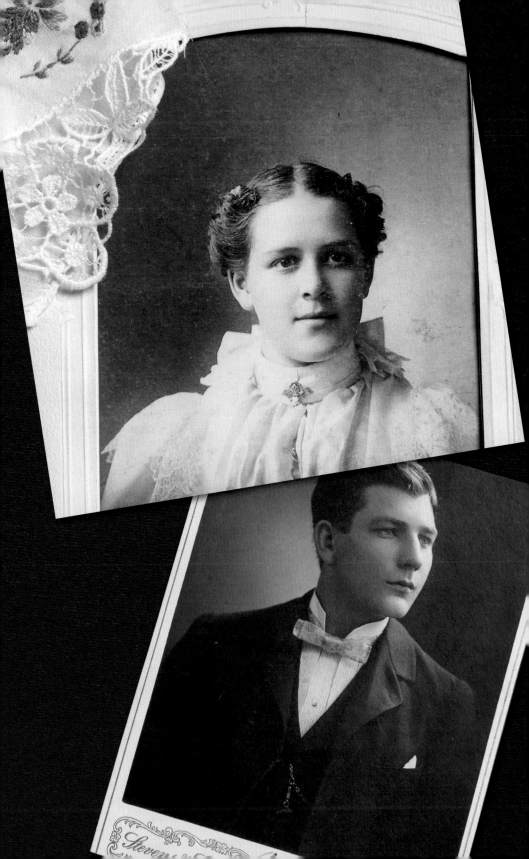

introduction. How was he going to meet her?

One day, it almost happened, though as fate would have it, the circumstances were all wrong. This story has been told in the Sartor family for more than a century.

Mary was in her family's backyard when she saw Pierre begin to make his way across their lawn, but — *Horrors!* — the servant who did the family's laundry was off that day and Mary's unexalted reason for being outside was to hang the wash on the clothesline. A first meeting under these conditions simply would not do, so as Pierre traipsed through their yard, Mary took refuge among the wet, flapping sheets, observing him from a distance.

Either Pierre was oblivious to the girl amid the laundry, or he didn't let her appearance bother him, because he kept finding reasons to walk through the Winandy family's yard on subsequent days. By now, however, he was under another person's gaze.

Mary was the oldest of six children. At the time, her mother, Mary Borst Winandy, a lady in chronic frail health, was having a difficult pregnancy. Like Pierre's sister Liss back in Luxembourg, Mary had taken on many responsibilities of caring for her siblings. Her younger brother, Alfred, looking out upon the lawn, would return the favor — while extending the drama of Pierre and Mary's courtship a bit longer.

One day Alfred called out to Pierre: *Say, haven't I seen you about, cutting through our yard?*

Pierre would never admit to being there with the intent to impress the young lady of the house. He chose his words with care: *Your house of flowers is like the home of my childhood. Luxembourg is my old country. I am here in medical school.*

My father emigrated from Luxembourg, the boy countered.

Their exchange continued and Alfred finally said: *Call me Freddie.* He invited Pierre inside the house. It was late afternoon — teatime. In his unaffected way, Freddie said: *My sister is smitten. With you.*

Freddie led Pierre into the tiled and glass-enclosed back porch, then through the kitchen with its black-and-white checkerboard floor; copper pans hung overhead. They made their way to the dining room and settled at the table, which was covered with a lace cloth. Fresh roses graced the room.

The Winandys had household staff, and one of the servants had set out afternoon tea. Freddie offered refreshments to Pierre and led the conversation. Only a boy, Freddie was at ease in the fine surroundings. Pierre was impressed. Eager to fit in, Pierre made sure that when he placed his cup in the saucer, it made not a sound.

Pierre began to wonder: *Where is the mother? The other children?* And, most important: *Where is Freddie's sister, the lovely daughter?*

Although this scene has been a cherished part of the Sartor family history since the 1890s, some important details are lost, which creates a beguiling sense of mystery. Why did Freddie choose this particular day to invite Pierre into the house?

The fact is that as Freddie and Pierre chatted in the dining room, Freddie knew that Mary was achingly close but — once again — hiding from Pierre. In an irony of timing, this afternoon, like the previous occasion, was the day off for the girl who did the laundry and other cleaning chores. Mary had again taken on her duties, this time scrubbing the kitchen floor, when Freddie brought Pierre into the house. As they passed through the kitchen into the dining room, Mary ducked under the kitchen table. She peeked at her brother and his guest through the stitched openings of the eyelet tablecloth.

Decades later, Mary would say (as is recorded on tape): "I was kind of ashamed and I just took my — I climbed under the kitchen table."

By then a long-married and devoted couple, Pierre and Mary would describe — and coyly contest — these details. Apparently, it was thrilling for Mary to watch Pierre without being seen. She especially remembered his long handlebar mustache and the way it moved when he spoke.

What was Freddie thinking? With the servant who did their washing and cleaning off duty, he had the freedom to come up with his own plans. Did he enjoy teasing his big sister, hosting the young man who'd caught her fancy when he knew Mary was in no position to meet him? Or was Freddie well-meaning in his effort to get Mary and Pierre together that day but clueless, as boys can be, about social niceties, and unaware that Mary would not want to meet Pierre while she scrubbed the floor? A third possibility is that Freddie was playing the man of the house, drawing Pierre into conversation to assess Pierre as a potential beau for his sister. In this scenario, Freddie would know full well that Mary would not join them; if Pierre passed muster, he could be invited back — if not, Freddie would keep them apart.

Whatever Freddie's motives, he took charge of the situation and found Pierre to be acceptable. Before Pierre said farewell, he and Freddie planned a return visit, and this time, Freddie would ensure Mary was ready. Pierre would again stroll through the Winandy yard between the residence and the greenhouse. Freddie would appear and, in the most proper way, introduce Pierre to his sister, Mary Magdalene. And so it happened.

Their almost-comedic close calls were finished. The next time he was invited into the house, Pierre found himself in the parlor, sitting in a wing chair near the fireplace. Mary, her loose curls pinned back, sat in a matching chair on the other side of the fireplace. Mr. and Mrs. Winandy stood on each side of her. The proprieties commenced.

They were all "Luxies," they informed each other. Mr. Winandy inquired after the state of their home country. Pierre told of his family and the farm. He also worked in a reference to his mother's girlhood home, the finest in the village.

A week later, Pierre pulled his top hat and cane out of his trunk. They would come in handy when he paid a call on Mary: Now he could be taller than she. Mary Magdalene was 5 feet, 10 inches in height, quite tall for a girl in her generation. Pierre stood 5 feet, 7½ inches, average to a bit small for a man of that time. The top hat gave him stature in height and dignity.

Pierre began to visit Mary each Sunday. The laughter of small children often floated into the parlor from upstairs. By the sound, he thought they were roller skating or giving one another rides in a wheelbarrow across the wooden floors above. Bouncing balls? Surely a jump rope tapped the floor. More than one nanny rushed past the pocket doors. Wooden heels thumped, as servants went up and down the back stairs, bringing treats and tending to the children.

As their relationship progressed throughout the autumn, Pierre fit into a comfortable pattern with the Winandy family. Permission was granted for Mary to receive Pierre alone in the parlor when he called upon her. Later in the visit, other members of the family would join them. There might be a piano recital, charades, a game of cards. Pierre was beginning to feel more at home at Mary's house than at Ferdinand's. Perhaps it was the big family, the chatter and clatter, the back and forth that is typical in a house full of children. In addition to Mary, who turned 16 that October, and Freddie, going on eight, Pierre got to know Regina, 11 years old; Susanna, nine; Michael, four; and Peter Henry, a toddler who amused them while learning to walk. Pierre enjoyed talking with their father, Michael. He rarely saw Mrs. Winandy, still "in delicate condition," as well-bred Victorians described pregnancy, but having lost his mother as a boy, he was accustomed to a lively family without the mother being present.

Christmas of 1895 approached. Pierre was invited to the tree lighting. This was a high honor, and a sign of his favored standing with the Winandys.

On December 24, the sun having set in late afternoon, Pierre waited with Mary's family as they gathered, hushed, in the spacious entrance hall of their home. A servant opened the doors to the parlor, and what to their wondering eyes did appear but a scene of pure enchantment: The Christmas tree stood tall, candles aglow, decked with strings of popcorn and tinsel strips that glittered in the flickering light.

Mary's father invited Pierre to return on Christmas Day. He would not need to bring a calling card to place in the silver tray in the vestibule at the front door. He would always be welcome.

When Pierre arrived next morning, the Christmas tree had become a cornucopia, its tiered limbs sheltering an astonishing array of gifts. A hobby horse . . . a chalkboard . . . a tin soldier . . . games and dolls . . . there was a profusion of toys for every age. A photo shows a large golden harp nestled in the Christmas tree branches.

Pierre had not been poor in Luxembourg. He certainly felt he had more than enough, but his experience with Christmas had been candy and fruit, usually accompanied by a handmade wooden toy. This was an abundance he had not imagined. Despite the differences in how their families celebrated the holiday, Pierre felt comfortable with the Winandys. He saw the nativity set, symbol of their shared faith. He saw relatives expressing love for one another. Those were the qualities, he knew, that mattered most.

As the hoopla quieted, Mary led Pierre to a corner of the parlor. She pulled a photograph album down from a high shelf and opened its heavy brass clasp. She turned one page, then the next. Each image was framed in a cardboard mat bearing the name of a respected professional photographer. Each photo told a story, and Pierre realized this was Mary's way of drawing him into her family. Pierre saw younger but recognizable faces of Mary's siblings. She showed him a picture of Albert, who was close to her age, but who had died of rabies six years before.

Pierre admired how Mary took care of the younger children. He was impressed that she was willing to fill in for the chore girl when necessary. She was willing to work, to go where she was needed, to make things right. She was also a young lady of grace and charm who shared his faith and, clearly, had set her cap for him.

Later, back at Ferdinand's house, Pierre talked about the lavish Christmas tree and the photo album. His brothers were

Christmas in the Winandy home was a festive time. It was a high honor for Pierre to be invited to join the family's celebration.

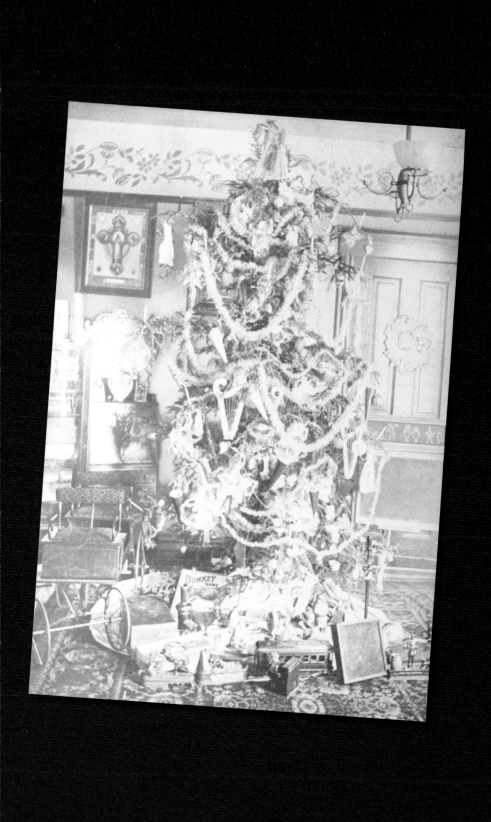

impressed. They knew Michael Winandy as the man who rented his greenhouses to them. Now their brother was courting Mr. Winandy's eldest daughter and was an honored guest in her home.

As time went on, in addition to visiting, Pierre sent letters to Mary; he liked to express himself in writing. Her letters have not survived, but we know of one in which she made clear her intent. It consists of just five words, delivered via the U.S. Postal Service:

Pierre,

Will you marry me?

And then came Pierre's last months of medical school. He reciprocated the intention that Mary had expressed.

Pierre asked Michael Winandy for his daughter's hand in marriage. Mary's father said yes.

But it would not be long before Pierre had yet another plan, which no one expected — least of all, Pierre himself.

Michael Winandy, Sr., a successful business leader in Chicago, gave his approval when Pierre asked for his daughter's hand in marriage — but he had misgivings about Pierre's plans for moving to Iowa.

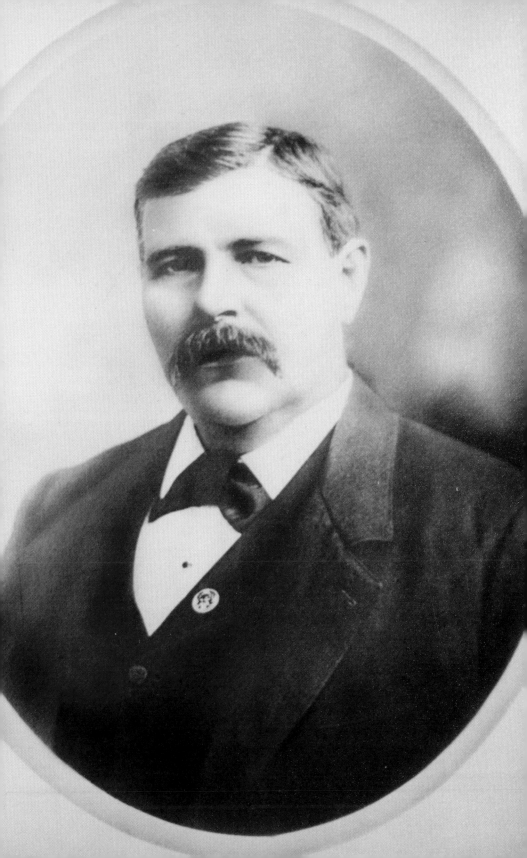

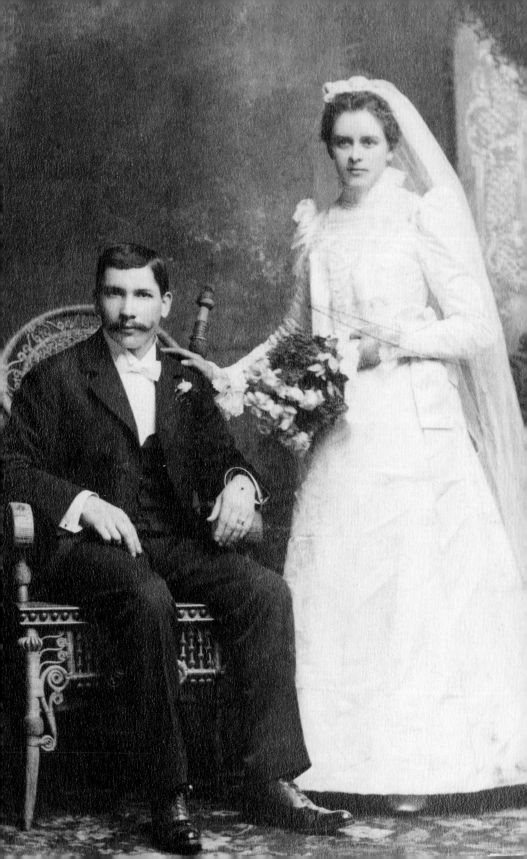

CHAPTER 8

Marriage and Career: Fulfillment and Frustration

Chicago, Illinois
1898-1900

THE BENNETT MEDICAL SCHOOL CLASS OF 1896 was scheduled to graduate on Tuesday evening, March 31. At some point in the winter or early spring, as Pierre contemplated his future — which now included being engaged — he met a medical student named John Klein at a social gathering. Their conversation set the direction for the rest of Pierre's life.

Klein was a Luxembourg-born pharmacist who had come to the United States to study medicine. While Pierre's ocean voyage was traumatic, Klein's trip afforded opportunities for social pleasantries. He became acquainted with a fellow passenger, John B. Mousel, who was returning to the United States from an extended visit with relatives in Luxembourg.

Mousel was the mayor of Bancroft, Iowa, a small town about 450 miles west of Chicago. He told Klein that a good number of people in his town were immigrants from Luxembourg and their descendants; many spoke German and were Catholic —

Devoted to their faith and to each other, Pierre and Mary were married on October 20, 1898 — her 19th birthday.

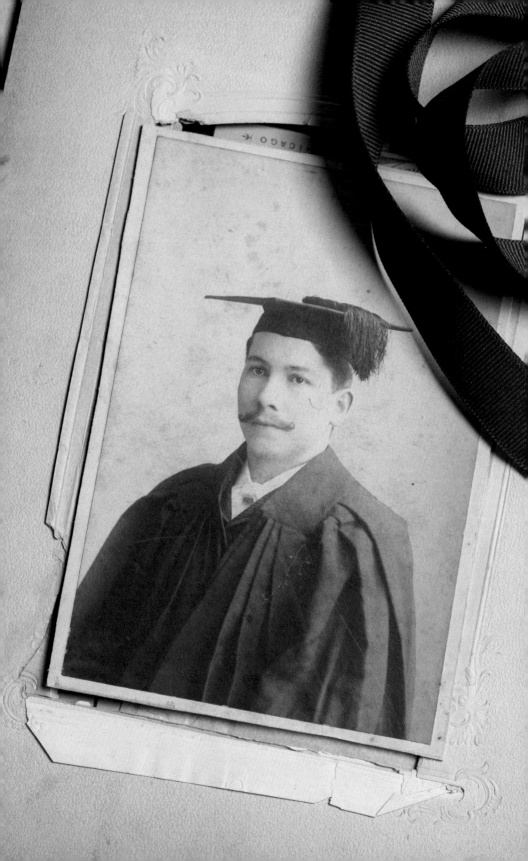

and Bancroft needed a doctor who could serve that population. Klein planned to remain in Chicago, but he thought Pierre might be interested . . .

Interested? Pierre was inspired.

In Chicago, Pierre knew, he would practice medicine in an office, day after day, with patients coming to him. In rural Iowa, he could roam, going from one patient to another, living the country life he knew as a boy in Luxembourg.

In a small town, Pierre would encounter the full range of medical conditions, not just the everyday sore throats and babies to deliver, which could fill up his practice in Chicago. He would see entire families, their relationships to one another and to others in the area. He would doctor an entire town. His sense of community was strong.

The Catholic dimension of Bancroft also appealed to Pierre. He enjoyed medical school and excelled at his studies, but never felt comfortable with the secularism he encountered from his first day. Pierre's calling to medicine was inseparable from his faith.

And Iowa was west of Chicago! Not the Wild West of Buffalo Bill, of course, but distant enough to kindle a young man's spirit.

It was an offer Pierre was highly inclined to accept.

The next day, he told Mary and her parents about this exciting opportunity. An awkward pause ensued. Eyes narrowing, Pierre's future father-in-law made it clear he knew no man named Klein and nothing of Iowa. The Winandy family, who had welcomed Pierre to their home with such warmth, now evinced an entirely different reaction to him.

I have to go. I am needed, Pierre said — and this became his mantra for life. He knew it the moment he said it.

Mary's father was disappointed. This idea meant that his eldest daughter would move far away, from the world-class city

Even before his graduation from medical school in Chicago, Pierre wanted to practice in rural Iowa.

that was her home to a remote prairie town.

Mary's mother collapsed. Well into her pregnancy, she already dreaded losing her engaged daughter's help with the younger children. And now this?

Back at home, Ferdinand and Francois were puzzled. Pierre had never been to the prairie. They hoped he would stay in one of the country's fastest-growing cities, where so many opportunities awaited. *The Chicago Medical Times* reported that of Pierre's class of 30 students, 18 had arranged to stay in the Chicago area.

They would be so proud to have their brother be a doctor — here, in their neighborhood. They had made it possible for Pierre to attend medical school. Yet from what Pierre was saying, the Sartors' togetherness would be short-lived. It seemed that Pierre wanted to get his diploma and be on his way.

In these painful conversations, one thing became clear: The wedding would be delayed. The decision was difficult, but Pierre accepted it. He wanted to settle this issue of practicing medicine on the prairie before he began a new life with Mary. He couldn't yet put into words what was drawing him west. Perhaps all could be resolved after he graduated in a few weeks. Under the circumstances, Pierre had to wonder: *Will Mary and her parents attend the ceremony?* She had already placed the invitation in the family's photo album.

The fraught conditions only became worse. The week before Pierre's graduation, Mary's new baby brother, John Valentine Winandy, was born on Monday, March 23. He died on Sunday, March 29, at the age of six days, barely 48 hours before Pierre was due to receive his diploma.

Now it was Mary's call to be needed — at home with her family. She was 16½, deeply in love and eager to be out of her parents' house. But she was held back by legitimate demands that kept her in place. She couldn't plan a wedding now, and her mother would be no assistance. Mary's life stalled.

Her intended had challenges of his own. Equally in love, Pierre was drawn to a future that would take Mary from everything she knew.

Graduation from medical school, so long awaited, was now upon him. Pierre must have thought of the mother who loved him . . . the father who sacrificed for him . . . the sisters who believed in him . . . the doctor who restored his hearing . . . the years of education and living on his own . . . the trip across the Atlantic . . . the brothers who cared for him in childhood illness and paved his way in America . . . the profession that was his calling . . . his classmates who were seizing opportunities that abounded . . . the Winandy family who made him one of their own . . . and the beautiful girl he hoped to marry.

As these thoughts churned, Pierre — described by *The Chicago Medical Times* as "one of the best" in his class — had no firm plans for his future.

Graduation was a gala event, covered in *The Chicago Medical Times*. Whether Mary and her family attended is not known. To Pierre it had to seem the pinnacle of his life thus far.

The ceremony included 350 guests, the largest crowd ever for Bennett Medical College. Pierre's class had the highest grade point average in the school's history, 91.9, and he was near the top.

Dr. Anson Clark, president and dean of the college, described the banquet as the "most brilliant and successful of any in the history of the college." Sweet music brightened the hum of conversation and the soft tread of waiters. It was an evening of great joy and gladness for the graduates.

In his address, Dr. Clark declared they were on the cusp of an explosion of medical knowledge. Pierre's class had already been introduced to the germ theory and laboratory-based training in bacteriology. Dr. Clark told the graduates that scientific progress was so rapid they would need to update their skills on an ongoing basis.

Soon they were singing their class song: "Through all the world we roam afar. . . ."

There were toasts, customized for various students. Pierre may have shared thoughts about his future since the toast in his honor had a distinctive Western theme: "Blisters and Saddle Sores."

A light spirit prevailed as the night of March 31 went on. At midnight, Professor J.B. McFatrich made an urgent announcement: *Please, a lady has lost a valuable silk handkerchief. Could all take a moment and search under the tables?*

The gallant young physicians dove under the tables, creating a humorous spectacle of well-tailored backsides thrust into the air . . . *April fools, my friends!* called out the jovial professor.

The clock — and the month — had just changed. It was April 1, 1896.

Pierre would always keep his diploma wrapped in brown paper, tied up with string, just the way it arrived from the Illinois State Board of Health. It is still in its wrap today, addressed to "Pierre Sartor, M.D., 4074 N. Clark St. — Station X, Collect."

He also kept a copy of the Physician's Prayer, which he had first seen on the wall of his doctor's office in Luxembourg.

With his engagement in flux and career plans unclear, Pierre's faith would be more important than ever. Immediately after graduation, he went into action and boarded a train from Chicago to Bancroft, Iowa.

We do not know exactly what his plans were in making the trip, and perhaps Pierre himself did not know, either. He was guided by the words of his father, Mathias Sartor, when he had left home to receive treatment for his ear condition: *First things first. As long as it takes.* This statement is decisive — yet in Pierre's actions at this point, there is an ambiguous quality to the words as well.

On one hand, Pierre's prompt departure after graduation suggests an exploratory trip — the chance to see for himself what the town of Bancroft and state of Iowa had to offer. In this case, he would be gone *as long as it takes* to make the decision if, indeed, this was the place where he would begin his medical career.

On the other hand, when Pierre's train stopped in Des Moines, he sought out the State Board of Medical Examiners to inquire about getting a license to practice medicine in Iowa. This indicates Pierre was more than a casual visitor; he was preparing to put down roots.

Both scenarios had the benefit of creating space for Pierre, given his recent awkwardness with the Winandy family. But creating space carried its own risk. Would Mary wait for him, or might he lose her? Communication is essential in any relationship, and it is especially important for engaged couples who are finding the way to create a shared path in life. Mary's definition of *as long as it takes* might have been quite different from Pierre's.

If Pierre thought the trip would help clarify his plans, he met disappointment at the first stop. There would be no license to practice medicine in Iowa at this point. The clerk was friendly enough but said the Board of Medical Examiners would not meet again for five months. As a result, when he got on the train to Bancroft, Pierre was heading away from home, family and fiancée, going to a place where he knew nobody, with no clear idea of what he would do or how long he would stay.

But the young doctor who had overcome childhood illness, absence from loved ones and a trip across the Atlantic Ocean took it all in stride.

Leaving Des Moines, Pierre's train passed into the countryside until he reached his destination about 150 miles north and slightly west, approaching the Iowa border with Minnesota. As a newspaper later described, "Sporting a sweeping black mustache and his brand-new medical degree, young Dr. Sartor went to Bancroft." The town was founded barely a decade before, in 1881, and named for George Bancroft (1800-1891), an American historian and diplomat.

Bancroft and Titonka, Pierre's later home, are located in Kossuth County, the largest county in the state of Iowa. The county is named for Lajos Kossuth (1802-1894), a Hungarian statesman and a powerful orator and writer who inspired followers in many places throughout the world.

It would not be until 1934 that Bancroft was termed "The Garden Spot of Iowa," but its rural charm won over Pierre. In a region of black loam and luxurious vegetation, the area was noted for its timber, rivers and creeks. Agriculture and family-owned businesses — several of them still in operation today

— formed the bedrock of the economy.

Nine years after it was first surveyed, Bancroft registered a population of 657 in the census of 1890. By the time Pierre arrived, the city was growing, rebuilding from a fire on December 13, 1893, that destroyed much of the downtown.

Pierre did not slip unobserved into town. On his first Sunday, he went to Mass, decked out in his Prince Albert coat and top hat — suitable attire, perhaps, for attendance at one of the socially prominent churches in Chicago, but out of place in Kossuth County, Iowa. Soon, several children were laughing and pointing at him.

The next day Pierre took to exploring and listing the features of Bancroft that Mary might appreciate. Its size and setting deeply appealed to him. From many places in town, he could see beyond the buildings into the countryside; it reminded him of his village in Luxembourg.

At the same time, there was a vibrancy to Bancroft far more attractive to Pierre than the place where he had grown up.

He saw well walls cemented, several hundred feet deep. Clear water! And, on Main Street, he found just the corner for his office. Never mind it was above the meat market. That meant plenty of people would pass by. It was also next to a tailor and a harness store, and across from a café. There was a grain business . . . a hardware store . . . a public school. A lawyer's shingle flapped in the breeze. Two drugstores. The volunteer fire brigade had a cart with a water tank, pump and whistle.

For recreation there was a box-ball alley, where friendly opponents played a game that was similar to four square. More enticing to youth, although less salubrious, was the Bancroft pool hall, an institution of small-town, turn-of-the-century Iowa made famous in the song "Ya Got Trouble" in stage and screen productions of *The Music Man*.

Pierre was one of the highest-ranked students in the Bennett Medical College Class of 1896.

A.

IOWA STATE BOARD OF HEALTH.

PHYSICIAN'S CERTIFICATE.

DIPLOMA

SCHOOL OF PRACTICE.

Eclectic

TO

Pierre Sartor

Dated *August 7th* 189*6.*

Filed for record the *26th* day

of *October* A. D. 189*6*

and recorded in Book of Certificates.

No. *1* Page *4*

M.S. Randall

County Recorder.

There was a Catholic church with a parochial school, a Methodist Episcopal church, a Swedish Lutheran church and a Baptist church. Pierre would have the support of these pillars of the community when he cared for the townspeople.

As a young man living on his own, Pierre also found his way to the saloon — after all, it was one of the best places to make oneself known and pick up the talk of the town. Pierre let it out that he was a doctor, and the locals regaled him with tales of his professional forebears.

Stories about Doc Cogley were legion, although more than 40 years had passed since Cogley came to Kossuth County. It was probably a form of hazing, but men at the bar relished telling young Pierre Sartor, M.D., with his cultured accent and European manners, how Doc was called to help a patient one day, name of Old Dutch Henry. The man's leg was frostbitten, stiff as a tree limb. Doc couldn't treat Old Dutch, so he sawed the man's leg off.

Pierre didn't blanch at these stories. In fact, he thrived in Bancroft. He trimmed his handlebar to the brush-style mustache that local men favored. He met people from Luxembourg, some of whose names were familiar to him from the old country.

Pierre also tended to his first patient. A man named Nolan was at the Phoenix Hotel. He was sick and, at this point, unconcerned about the rules and regulations of the Iowa State Board of Medical Examiners. Pierre lacked a license, but it must have been a positive encounter. He earned his first dollar as a practicing physician and put it in a frame.

It's not clear if Pierre saw other patients during the three months he was in Bancroft. By all evidence he was putting down roots, biding his time until he could get his license and open his practice. He befriended a local physician, Dr. C.R. Cretzmeyer, who more than half a century later would introduce Pierre to audiences who honored Pierre's career-long medical service. On those occasions in the far future, Dr. Cretzmeyer would say of Pierre: "He came to Bancroft . . . where I first met him and can still number him among my best friends . . . a hale fellow well met."

Then a letter came from Chicago. Dr. Lentes, the physician in High Ridge who cared for Pierre's brothers' families and had endorsed Bennett for his medical education, was dead. The Sartor families, Mary's family and the other people in High Ridge who had been so welcoming to Pierre now needed a doctor.

Pierre had to reconsider. His Iowa license was in the future and the situation in Chicago was immediate, pressing. His professional mantra now sent him in an unexpected direction, back to High Ridge.

I am needed, he told his new friends in Iowa. *I must return.*

This decision had the great benefit of reuniting Pierre with Mary. He was so excited to see her again. But inside, Pierre knew. A small town would always hold his heart. For him it would be Berbourg and Bancroft.

On his way back to Chicago, passing again through Des Moines, Pierre purchased a leather journal, a honey-hued beauty. It would cover the three months that he determined would elapse before he could secure his license to practice medicine in Iowa. He wrote in a new date every half page.

Pierre returned to Chicago in the summer of 1896, almost three years after he first arrived in High Ridge. The summer was busy from the start.

While Pierre was out walking one day, a wild-eyed fireman leaped into his path. The man begged — *Please come to my house!* He talked fast, in a clipped Chicago accent. He pulled Pierre by the sleeve to his home around the corner, and before long the new doctor had delivered, as he wrote by hand on the letterhead stationery of his practice, a "19-pound baby."

The birth registry went straight to his lockbox. He considered the event symbolic, a milestone in his career, and had a business card made showing a photo of a large-size infant.

Once Pierre's office was established in the neighborhood around Clark Street and Devon Avenue, he ran a tight and regular schedule, seven days a week. He was so busy that he lived in rented rooms above his office.

Pierre's journal shows that his first scheduled appointment

Wednesday

50.

Thursday 28

was with Mary's uncle, John Winandy, brother of her father, Michael. John Winandy had nothing wrong that Pierre could diagnose — except a pointed curiosity about the future of his niece. John told Pierre that Mary was hard at work at home, tending the children, supporting her mother.

We don't know if Pierre and Mary saw each other privately after he returned to High Ridge, but the account has survived of his first visit to her home. With Pierre sensing there might be a strain in his relationship with the family, he was prepared to signal formality by leaving his calling card. But, instead, he was welcomed and ushered into the parlor.

At last, Mary Magdalene entered the room. She untied her apron and greeted Pierre. Their future hung in the balance. Their exact words have not come down to us, but by all accounts, they resumed where they had left off. The separation had confirmed what Pierre and Mary both knew: They were in love.

Left unspoken were some important particulars, such as the date of their wedding and where they would live.

On many levels, Pierre was torn.

He wanted to practice in small-town Iowa but felt obliged to meet the need for medical care in Chicago.

He wanted to get married but doing so would tie him further to his wife's city.

While drawn to Bancroft, he also had a scientific bent and natural curiosity that attracted him to the educational opportunities of a major urban setting. Pierre applied to Cook County Hospital for an intensive six-month program, followed by a three-month surgical residency at St. Elizabeth's Hospital. In the milieu of rapidly advancing medical knowledge, Pierre relished his association with premiere physicians and the opportunity to care for patients with complex medical needs.

Another, more subtle, conflict entered Pierre's thinking. In

Pierre's journal records his busy practice in Chicago, but he was dissatisfied with urban life.

this sophisticated, metropolitan area, his medical skills and winning personality positioned him for success. He could become a "society doctor" with a highly remunerative practice.

But the drive was not there.

Pierre worked for a year on Clark Street. According to his diary, appointments of any kind were a dollar, recorded in pencil, one page for each day. He charged $10 for the difficult delivery of a baby, which happened frequently. Despite the fee structure that he carefully worked out, in the end, Pierre let everything depend on the patient's ability to pay.

He would never labor over his ability to earn money, not with any gusto. In time he realized: He was not fond of collecting.

Pierre's personal background compounded the issue. He sought social and economic advancement in coming to America — but now that he could earn money, he was reluctant to ask patients to pay when their finances were a problem.

As time went by in his Chicago practice, something else nagged. Patients in the big city lived stacked one floor above another, in tall buildings. Should a contagious disease ever come, even a dedicated physician like Dr. Sartor would be daunted in the hope of providing meaningful care.

Pierre was busy — yet unfulfilled. *They do not know me very well.*

He had more to give.

When accepting the call to High Ridge, Pierre promised himself it would last three months, but almost before he knew it, two years had passed, with no end in sight. Mary's mother was pregnant again. Mrs. Winandy was frail; her eldest daughter — Pierre's fiancée — was under more obligation than ever to provide support at home.

Deliverance came from a familiar, yet unexpected, source. John Klein, the man who had told Pierre of the opening in

While attending patients in his Clark Street office, Pierre undertook advanced training at the prominent hospitals and surgical clinics of Chicago.

COOK COUNTY HOSPITAL

Admit Mr.

Student of

Expiring October 1, 1896

Bancroft, Iowa, back in the spring of 1896, was now set to graduate from medical school. A thought occurred to Pierre: Could Klein take his place as the doctor for High Ridge? In their conversations, Pierre extolled the virtues of a busy practice in a well-to-do community with the advantages of a leading city nearby.

The moment? *Ripe.*

Klein agreed.

Pierre became a man with a plan. With a successor lined up for his High Ridge practice, he and Mary could set a date for their wedding. They chose October 20, 1898. This was symbolic — Mary's 19th birthday. To Pierre, the date was also strategic. It provided a window of time for him to go to Des Moines and secure his Iowa medical license, followed by a visit to Bancroft to arrange his office there. After the wedding, he and Mary could make a seamless transition to their new home.

Back in Chicago, his Iowa medical license in hand, Pierre checked off the days. His presence was a sign of reassurance to the bride's family. Most important, he and Mary were about to enter into Holy Matrimony, one of the seven sacraments that were the cornerstone of their Catholic faith.

At last, he turned the journal to October 20, 1898, which he had marked with a ribbon.

On the prescribed hour, in his top hat and Prince Albert coat, Pierre arrived at St. Henry Church, the church his brothers' families attended and which he had seen soon after arriving in High Ridge.

Mary and her bridesmaids arrived first: Missy Muno, Mary's friend since childhood, and Regina, Mary's younger sister.

Mary's parents, her mother in advanced pregnancy, arrived next, in a carriage. Pierre sympathized with the challenges that Mary's mother faced. Her frequent pregnancies and the care of her large family were draining, and now the wedding of her eldest daughter was upon her.

Mary's brothers were in the row. To help maintain decorum, the younger boys had helpers positioned between them. Mary's other sister, Susanna, was also in the mix.

Pierre absorbed the elegance around him. Michael Winandy must have emptied his greenhouses for this event.

When approaching the church, Pierre had seen flower petals on the sidewalk and street. As he looked around the sanctuary, there were blossoms including roses and gladiolas atop wicker stands, over the doorways and at the altar. The men wore boutonnieres in their lapels and the ladies had delicate floral arrangements on their shoulders. Many of the adult women wore orchids, a rare and expensive flower.

Pierre stood at the altar, shoulder to shoulder with his best man, Dominick Geymer, a pharmacist, class of '98. Next to him was Pierre's groomsman, his brother Ferdinand.

Pierre looked down the flower-strewn aisle as Mary Magdalene stepped into the archway of the vestibule, still in shadows. And then the organ played one of those chords that stretch a moment to infinity.

Mary started up the aisle, escorted by her father. Pierre was shaken by the vision of her coming toward him, the most beautiful sight he had ever seen. It was as though he stood in a snow globe, surrounded by the colors, the light and the flowers.

Mary carried her First Communion prayer book, bound in ivory and trimmed in mother-of-pearl. In years to come, Pierre and Mary's daughters and their daughter-in-law, my mother, Luella, would carry the same book on their wedding day. Mary carried it again when she and Pierre renewed their vows on their golden wedding anniversary in 1948.

Pierre and Mary exchanged vows and the Nuptial Mass ended. Pierre was looking forward to the reception where wine from Luxembourg would flow, and there would be music and dancing.

But the celebration got started early. The sounds of music, marching and cheering echoed into the church. There was a parade outside, perhaps a patriotic rally associated with the Spanish-American War then underway. The country was about to enter what Henry Luce of *Time* magazine would later call "The American Century." It seemed an auspicious start to their marriage.

There was good news within the family, too. A month after the wedding, Mary Magdalene's mother delivered a new baby, whom they named Thomas Pierre Winandy. The baby lived and Pierre felt proud and honored that his new brother-in-law carried his name.

For Pierre, marriage to Mary Magdalene brought joy — but professionally, he was not where he wanted to be. The near-miss pattern of their early courtship now manifested itself in his career.

After the wedding, there was no departure for Iowa. Although Pierre had his license to practice there, he and Mary continued to live in Chicago. The reasons are not clear, but the situation was compounded by the fact that within five months after getting married, Mary was expecting a baby. Their daughter, Mary Catherine, whom they called May, was born on December 28, 1899. She had dark hair and fair skin and, it was said, was just as beautiful as all the Winandy babies.

With fatherhood following soon after marriage, Pierre had more responsibilities than ever. But he never lost his dream of his home on the prairie. If Mary was distressed with his idea, we don't know of it. Apparently, Mary looked forward to the adventure of mothering just one child, their own.

Being a father strengthened Pierre's resolve. So did the knowledge that Mary, unlike her mother, was healthy and strong during pregnancy and following delivery. They could make it on their own, as a couple and as a young family.

One day, soon after May was born, Pierre and Mary called on her parents. It was only her father who met them in the parlor. Pierre said, in as few words as possible, what amounted to this: He would move the Winandys' firstborn, and their only grandchild, to the Iowa prairie. Full well he knew — he braced himself — that he was taking the eldest daughter away from

Mary Magdalene Winandy carried her First Communion prayer book on her wedding day, as have other brides in the author's family for more than a century.

136

Mary Magdalena
Hinandy
(Mrs. Pierre
Sartor)
1st Communion
Prayerbook

Chicago, Ill.
1892.

born 1879
died nov 13 1912

born 1898 9

written by L M Sartor

her family. But he wanted to go where his medical skills would be best used. Where his fluency in German would be an asset. He would be a Catholic doctor to a town of many Catholics.

This cannot have been a surprise to Mr. Winandy; the topic had been rumbling around in the family since Pierre and Mary's engagement, before his graduation from medical school. Given the passage of time, Mr. Winandy likely hoped that Pierre would settle into life in Chicago, particularly now that he was a husband and father. Mary's presence and obvious support strengthened Pierre's case, but the strained conversation fell into its old, familiar pattern. The hour in the Winandy parlor seemed like a decade.

That is when a new dynamic changed the picture. Mrs. Winandy — Mary's near-invalid mother — assumed, for the first time in Pierre's relationship with the family, a dominant role. To Pierre, it seemed she stepped out of the shadows, and her message was clear: She was the new grandmother — they had a baby to baptize — and the baby needed a gown!

As with Christmas and the wedding, the Winandys' way of doing things was attractive to Pierre, but a bit overwhelming. They approached the sacrament of baptism with gusto.

Mary Magdalene had her own baptismal gown, which had sufficed for her siblings. But it was cotton, reflecting the family's financial standing some two decades before, and that would not do for Mrs. Winandy's granddaughter. May must be swathed in silk organza with Alençon lace from France.

Known as the "Queen of Lace," Alençon originated in its namesake community west of Paris in the 17th century; today, like the dancing procession of Echternach, in which Pierre had participated as a boy in Luxembourg, this type of lace is recognized on the UNESCO Representative List of the Intangible Cultural Heritage of Humanity.

His mother-in-law's edict stirred a memory for Pierre. On the French tramp steamer that took him to America, Pierre had seen crates of Alençon lace. The crew members were far more solicitous of this cargo than they were of the immigrant passengers. During his voyage in 1893, the lace was near to Pierre but impossibly out of reach. Six years later, his daughter would wear it.

Mrs. Winandy took Mary in hand for an expedition to Marshall Field's, the Chicago institution for luxury shopping. The first of its iconic clocks had recently been installed at the corner of State and Washington Streets. May's lace baptismal gown is part of our family's collection. It has done service for other babies in our family over the past century.

The baptism was held at St. Henry in the holiday season of 1899, the church filled with poinsettias from Michael Winandy's greenhouses. Family and friends attended the service, followed by a reception at the grandparents' spacious home.

It was a milestone occasion, but Pierre was looking ahead. He even committed his plans to writing. His diary from this time bears the statement that he would leave for Iowa at the end of December; Mary and the baby would follow at the end of January.

And yet, once again, it was not to be.

Pierre, Mary and the baby stayed another year in Chicago. There is no evidence that Pierre wavered in his desire to relocate to Iowa or that Mary opposed the plan. Other factors, including the demands of everyday living, must have been at work. The months ticked by.

For reasons we do not know, Pierre finally made the break from Chicago. He went to Bancroft to set up his practice. It was November 1900. Pierre and Mary had been married for two years; baby May was approaching her first birthday.

Now the plans fell into place, and this time, at last, it all went smoothly. Pierre was back in High Ridge for Christmas. He hired workers to pack their belongings and purchased tickets for the train ride west. The little family would depart in January 1901, making a fresh start in the new year.

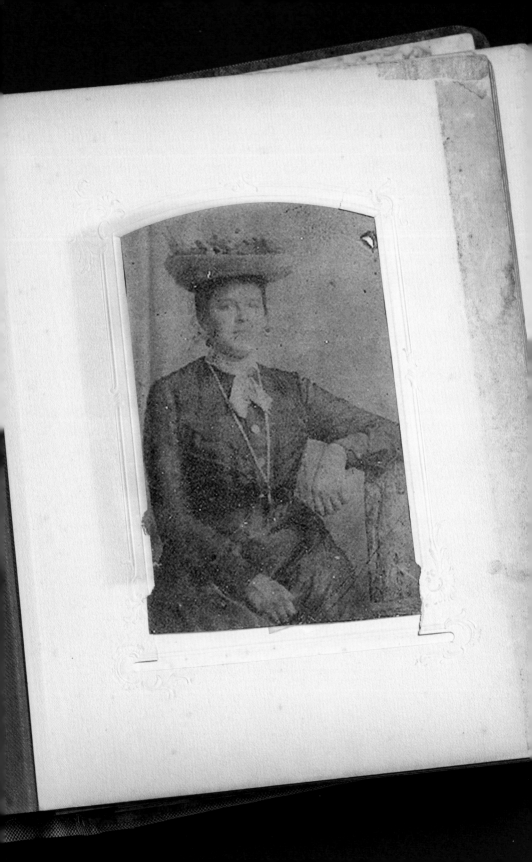

CHAPTER 9

A New Home

Bancroft, Iowa
1901

PIERRE AND MARY SETTLED THEMSELVES AND BABY MAY on the train. Then they headed back to the open caboose to wave goodbye. Friends and family clustered around the track, calling out their farewells.

The train's baggage car bulged with Mary's trunks. She also had hatboxes, satchels and bags and a special case for traveling on a train. Pierre's clothes and, importantly, his medical supplies, were packed as well.

The car was dark; it had aisles of blackened, greased wood. The countryside flashed by through the small windows. Soon the fields that Pierre had described to Mary flickered by the window. They were not gold as in his enthusiastic reports but, rather, covered in snow.

The train stopped at various stations. Pierre and Mary observed women wrapped in shawls, farmers in rough coats,

Pierre wondered if his young wife, with her refined upbringing and monogrammed luggage, would adjust to living in a small town. He needn't have worried.

their faces weathered and cold.

Mary had not seen anything like this. As a child, she had been to the train station in Chicago, and she'd worn her best frock. Her mother wore a mantle, a sleeveless tailored long cloak. In Mary's world, one dressed up to travel and to receive guests as they arrived.

At a stop along the way, Mary got out to have a look. Her report: The little room in the station smelled like wet wool coats.

Pierre and Mary had talked about moving to Iowa for years. By all accounts, and by the support she showed for Pierre when he raised the subject with her parents, she supported the plan. However, now that they were actually making the move, Pierre must have wondered if Mary, with her refined upbringing and monogrammed luggage, would adjust to the small-town, rural life he so eagerly sought. Gamely, he promised she would get her pep back when she saw their new home.

It was not long after when Pierre discovered something that helped assure him Mary had the fortitude required for such a change in living conditions. She was napping with baby May in her arms. A low sun shone through the window and Pierre caught a flash of silver glinting near Mary's ankle. Pierre jumped to his feet.

His wife had a pistol strapped to her leg! He roused her to ask what this meant.

Father said I need it, Mary murmured, not yet fully awake.

Pierre had loved Mary since she was an adolescent, and he thought he knew his wife well, but this revelation took his admiration to a new level. There was a gutsy quality to Mary Magdalene Winandy Sartor, and Pierre began to relax about her adjustment to life on the prairie. Pierre realized it mattered a lot to him.

Mary Magdalene was Annie Oakley, his beloved wife and mother of his child all in one! He would entertain himself with that image for the rest of his life.

When they arrived in Bancroft, Pierre was proud to show off their new home, set within a generous front yard. It had cream clapboards and forest-green trim. The porch stood almost at ground level. They could push the baby's pram right into the house.

Mary waited inside the entry for her rocking chair to be unloaded. To the downstairs bedroom it went, where it would always stay. When the chair arrived, she settled into it. Windows of tiny panes surrounded her in this house of great light.

Pierre's earlier visits to Bancroft paid dividends. He had built up a circle of acquaintances and the arrival of a new doctor for the town, with a pretty wife and baby daughter to boot, attracted attention. Neighbors came in carts and buggies and on foot, bringing greetings and offering to help Doc and his family. The scene was more cordial than "Iowa Stubborn," in which the townspeople introduce themselves in *The Music Man*:

> *Oh, there's nothing halfway*
> *About the Iowa way to treat you*
> *When we treat you*
> *Which we may not do at all*
> *There's an Iowa kind of special*
>   *chip-on-the-shoulder attitude*
> *We've never been without*
> *That we recall.*

In fact, the Sartors' front door was filled for a long time. Pierre seemed to be greeting the entire town, Mary would say. Eventually, the bustle dwindled; the parade of visitors ended. The silence must have been exquisite after the long journey and moving in.

Pierre looked around — *Where was Mary?* Her rocking chair was empty.

The scene that came next is part of Sartor family lore.

Pierre made his way through the jumble of boxes, satchels, bags and trunks, searching for his wife. *Was she all right? Why had she gone off by herself?* He didn't see her. Anxiety rose: He wanted her to be happy here. Was the town, the house, a disappointment to her? Pierre pushed his way into the dining room, shouldering around boxes and crates, heading toward the kitchen at the back of the house.

143

Pierre paused — and his heart stopped. There, on the window seat in the dining room, framed in the bay window that glowed with soft light from the late afternoon, was Mary Magdalene. She held, with exquisite poise, a teacup and saucer from her wedding china. His wife might have been sitting for a portrait except, in a most attractive way, her hair was shaken down.

Pierre took in the scene. Mary had buttoned a fresh white collar and cuffs on her dress. An open trunk served as the table; it was her bridal hope chest. The sides of the chest were adorned with lithographs of elegant ladies depicted among bouquets of flowers. They seemed to join Mary at her tea party.

And perhaps most endearing of all, Mary had slipped off her shoes. On their first day in Bancroft, she was already at home.

Pierre joined her. They talked quietly, but most of the time they simply enjoyed each other's company. The baby slept.

For the rest of his life, the memory of that scene gave Pierre great joy. If he had feared Mary might think she'd left heaven behind when they moved to the prairie . . . no . . . heaven seemed to follow Mary wherever she went.

Within a week, the new home was arranged. It was also stuffed to the rafters with fresh flowers, posted from High Ridge, courtesy of Mary's father. In spring she could start a garden of her own. The phlox would grow so tall. And she would dry the lavender to place upon their sheets throughout the year.

The garden would be Mary's refuge. And the fresh breeze would flutter the linens and garments on her clothesline to the rhythm of the backyard water pump.

A meal served at home — that would have to wait. Mary had to find a house girl. Meanwhile, it was the custom for new residents to take meals at a boardinghouse nearby. Mary knew that supper would be the only occasion when she was likely to see Pierre. A small-town doctor would be on call — and in demand — most of the time.

But the right helper would be easy to find. Immigrants were willing to work for a family for food and board, she told Pierre.

I am an immigrant, Pierre reminded her, and he would say this, not often, but for the rest of his life.

Soon he filled out the form and became a United States citizen.

Mary found a young woman to help with chores, whose name has been lost. They became more than employer and maid. They were friends. She and Mary were the only adults in the house during waking hours. They set a pattern of doing household chores, taking care of May and having sociable visits.

During Pierre and Mary's first weeks in Bancroft, over dinner at the boardinghouse and later at home, Mary shared her discoveries of the town. After doing his best to promote Bancroft to her for several years, Pierre now came to see the town through Mary's eyes. He listened to every detail. The drugstore had a jewelry department! It also sold Native crafts.

There was a tailor shop, which Mary noted with special care. Getting Pierre to wear trousers of the proper length was a challenge and would be throughout their marriage. The young man at this shop, deftly using his needle, would be her ally.

Mrs. T.M. Ludwig managed a café. Mary pulled up a stool at the fountain and unpinned her hat for a breather.

Speaking of hats, Susie Hackl ran the millinery shop. Mary picked a new hat for the season. It had lavender flowers and grosgrain ribbons. Susie would deliver it in a case.

O.L. Harper, the photographer! The studio had chairs padded in velvet, and a watercolor backdrop depicting columns and flower baskets.

She did need to find the library — Where was the library? She would sign on as a volunteer.

While Pierre had recounted the business and recreational aspects of Bancroft to Mary (although how much he shared of the pool hall and saloon we do not know), and while Mary extolled the town's cultural and commercial features to him, it is significant that Pierre and Mary each saved their highest praise for St. John the Baptist Church and its parochial school. In session for the first time that year, it was located just past the edge of town looking toward the prairie, which beckoned to them both.

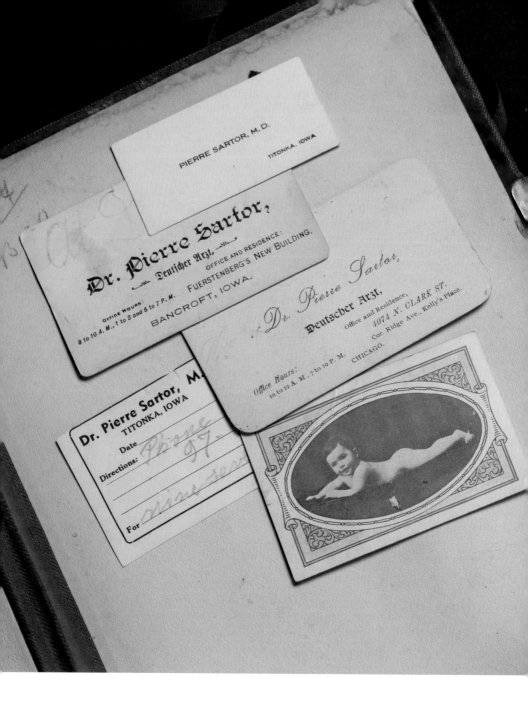

PIERRE SARTOR, M. D. TITONKA, IOWA

Dr. Pierre Sartor,
— Deutscher Arzt, —
OFFICE AND RESIDENCE:
FUERSTENBERG'S NEW BUILDING,
OFFICE HOURS:
8 to 10 A. M., 1 to 3 and 5 to 7 P. M.   BANCROFT, IOWA.

Dr. Pierre Sartor,
Deutscher Arzt,
Office and Residence:
4074 N. CLARK ST.
Cor. Ridge Ave., Kelly's Place.
Office Hours:
10 to 12 A. M., 7 to 10 P. M.   CHICAGO.

Dr. Pierre Sartor, M.
TITONKA, IOWA
Date
Directions:
For

Business cards chart the evolution of Pierre's career. Pierre chose a card depicting a hefty infant to commemorate his delivery of a 19-lb. baby.

CHAPTER 10

Calling Dr. Sartor

Bancroft, Iowa
1901-1918

PIERRE'S FAMILY THRIVED IN BANCROFT. At last Pierre had found the personal and professional environment he craved. A friend recalled: "He was as cheerful a neighbor as I remember having. No matter what the weather, snow, rain or 'slush,' at 'twenty-nine below' or 'ninety-nine above,' he always brightened the day with a cheerful smile."

In the evenings, Pierre would stroll down Main Street to his office, sit at his desk and mull over the day's events. Writing was a form of release, as satisfying to Pierre as music. He found that keeping a journal helped structure his thoughts while providing freedom to express himself at will. There was familiar comfort in the scratch of his pen over the onionskin paper, the scent of ink from the open well.

He recorded the challenges and satisfactions of being a small-town doctor in turn-of-the-century America. When he traveled on horseback, Pierre loaded up his saddlebags with what he thought the patient needed. On house calls, he carried his doctor bag from Chicago with its rounded lid containing a shelf for bottles in green, brown and clear glass. Pierre had Epsom salts to relieve pain and stiffness, or to coax splinters from the skin. Castor oil helped constipation and barley flushed toxins out of the kidneys. Pierre found that rural doctoring amounted to a lot of baby deliveries, typhoid and farm accidents. On November 1, 1907, the newspaper reported that a girl known as "Little Miss Ida May" had broken "her left thighbone last Thursday while playing on a straw pile . . . Dr. Sartor was called and set the fracture."

Pierre reached out to others when he needed help. A nurse in town was his capable assistant. The man who drove his horses could deliver anesthetic for an amputation.

Fastidious in all aspects of his life, especially his medical practice, Pierre had a sterilizer. He put it to frequent use for his instruments.

Pierre also counted on another device — the potbellied stove — as an essential tool in his medical practice. He knew that a friendly chat by the fire would relieve anxiety for many patients and their families. Although he lacked specialized training in conditions of mental and emotional distress, Pierre offered common sense, respect and empathy to patients with those conditions. According to a neighbor:

> I think one of Dr. Sartor's secrets is in the way in which he keeps secret the confidences of those whose burdens he shares. And as one thinks of his long hours at office, and in homes far and near, and as one thrills at the youthful buoyancy in his smile, his wit, his clothing, his sprightly step . . . one is pleased to share his spiritual tonics of interest in life, zest and faith.

One night, he received a frantic summons to a meeting of the Hesperian Society, a group dedicated to promoting good health in the community. The program had promised a fine entertainment. What went wrong?

The keynote speaker had come onstage before his large audience — and stopped breathing! He was in a state of collapse by the time Pierre reached him. Pierre did a careful evaluation. Diagnosis: Severe case of stage fright.

Hand-holding was the treatment, according to the story in

our family. The patient recovered.

As a physician, Pierre was welcome wherever he went. He was respected by all and beloved by many. But there was one form of treatment his patients resisted: surgery. *The people just don't believe in it*, he said. In the newspapers of the area, it was a common description to say a person "submitted to" an operation — language that conveyed the widespread belief that surgery was a last resort for patients in dire straits.

This was frustrating to Pierre and became more so as time passed. He found himself in an ironic situation. For years while living in Chicago, he had thought about, talked about, the virtues of practicing medicine in a rural community. Now that he was in Bancroft, he wanted to deliver the quality of care commensurate with his European education, big-city medical training, surgical residency at Cook County Hospital and postgraduate surgical training at St. Elizabeth's Hospital. He knew how to wield a scalpel and other surgical instruments, control bleeding and tie sutures. He had an atomizer to purify the air and create antiseptic conditions for optimal results.

A stickler for cleanliness, Pierre made the hygiene of his patients' homes a key part of his practice. A brief selection of references from the Board of Health shows his diligence:

> *Dr. Pierre Sartor fumigating Longergan, Mayer,*
> *Pearson & Odell homes*
> *Dr. Pierre Sartor disinfecting Stauftner house*
> *Dr. Pierre Sartor disinfecting Elbeck house*
> *Dr. Pierre Sartor disinfecting Bergman house*

Pierre followed medical news in the wider world. He was inspired by the work of Walter Reed in Cuba. The U.S. Army pathologist and bacteriologist conducted experiments showing that yellow fever is transmitted by the bite of a mosquito.

Pierre longed to make a difference, not on the scale of Walter Reed, but by delivering the best care he could to his patients. "I could diagnose," he wrote in his memoir, seeking ways to incorporate the research and knowledge of others into his practice.

Expanding his practice, Pierre applied to the Kossuth County Board of Supervisors to care for the indigent, a term for people in desperate poverty. Kossuth County was the largest county in Iowa, and Pierre was awarded the contract for the northern half: six towns and 14 townships. By horse and buggy, it took a great deal of time to see patients across this vast territory.

The benefits of this outreach would become manifest during the 1918 influenza pandemic. By providing care for widely scattered patients, Pierre learned the territory well. He would draw upon that knowledge amid the pressure of a health crisis to care for all his people.

And it didn't take but a few welcome-home hugs before Mary could identify the ethnic groups that Pierre had visited on any given day. He brought home their kitchen smells. For his part, Pierre said kitchen aromas were better than the formaldehyde that enveloped him during medical school.

Established in town, his skills in demand throughout half of the largest county in the state, Pierre continued to push himself. He still wanted his patients to accept surgery when their medical needs warranted it. The nearest hospital was in Algona, about 15 miles away — too far for procedures that could be done at home . . . for that matter, at his home.

There is perhaps no better example of the teamwork between Dr. and Mrs. Sartor than the fact that Mary Magdalene, who had grown up amid affluence and refinement, turned her kitchen into an operating room.

They called it Tonsil Tuesday and the word spread fast. Infected, inflamed tonsils were common among people of the time. Removal brought relief and helped folks adjust to the idea that surgery, when done properly, could be safe and beneficial. *By golly, Ma has the cleanest table in the county — perfect for operating on!* said Pierre, making the case to his prospective patients. His wife took this as high praise.

What one might think of as Pierre and Mary's zealous commitment to cleanliness became a family trait. Their son, my father, Guido, certainly inherited it. At dinner he wore a bib to protect his necktie and he insisted that all cloths — my mother's apron, the napkins, the dish towels, everything — had to be washed after each use. I remember when my mother, exasperated, finally asked him, *Do you think we have full-time help working in the laundry room?*

Pierre and Mary practiced what we would call holistic care. Their homey environment was reassuring to patients. With his European accent, and his confident and earnest manner, Pierre had a natural ability to put people at ease. Before the operation and afterward, as the patient awoke from anesthetic, Mary played the Victrola, cranking the handle and placing the needle on the phonograph. Musical selections might be the lilting Strauss waltzes that originated in Europe or the snappy Tin Pan Alley tunes of America. To recuperate, the patient would rest on a cot in the Sartors' bedroom by the front door or, in good weather, on the porch. Family and friends were welcome to stop by and escort the patient home.

Truth was, performing surgery at home helped Pierre as well as his patients. He needed time with his family, even if it was filtered through his professional responsibilities. The telephone at home rang around-the-clock. Pierre's mantra, to go where he was needed, kept driving him harder.

His sense of humor helped. He enjoyed telling this story:

Pierre implored one of his patients, an anxious mother: *Why, why do you always call me at night?*

But, Doctor, she helpfully explained, *you're so busy during the day!*

Pierre made progress in advocating for surgery. Tonsil Tuesday helped build credibility for surgical procedures, and his patients read newspaper and magazine accounts about successful operations in big cities. A new quandary then arose: Pierre could diagnose health problems that would respond to surgery — his patients were increasingly willing to have an operation — but a town the size of Bancroft could not support a hospital with the sophisticated services that his patients required.

In finding the solution, Pierre's mindset and the training of his alma mater served him well. Bennett Medical College's "eclectic" philosophy of seeking best practices reinforced Pierre's quest for excellence, which was the foundation of his entire career.

Timing and location aligned well for Pierre. He had access to the Algona Hospital in Iowa and St. Joseph Hospital in Mankato, Minnesota. Later in his career he had close associations with Park Hospital in Mason City, Iowa, where his son, my father, Dr. Guido Sartor, practiced.

In addition, barely 130 miles northeast of Bancroft was another small-town medical practice, but it was drawing physicians and patients from throughout the country and, indeed, around the world. Dr. William J. Mayo (Dr. Will) and his brother, Dr. Charles H. Mayo (Dr. Charlie), with their associates in Rochester, Minnesota, would become colleagues and friends of Pierre, establishing a personal and professional bond with the Sartor family that continues today, more than a century later.

There were many points of connection. Like Pierre, Dr. William Worrall Mayo — the father of Dr. Will and Dr. Charlie — was an immigrant. W.W. Mayo was born near Manchester, England, in 1819 and, like Pierre, as a young man in his 20s, made an ocean voyage to America. W.W. and Pierre were both of short stature — W.W.'s nickname was "the little doctor." They shared a strong sense of integrity, compassion for the poor and a commitment to excellence. Both physicians also exhibited what the Mayo family called a "questing spirit," a way to describe the restlessness that drove them west until they settled in their respective small, isolated Midwestern towns. W.W. Mayo was "a perfectionist who was readily infuriated by sloppy or second-rate work and was always delighted at any opportunity to improve medicine." The same could be said of Pierre.

The Mayo brothers were older contemporaries of Pierre, Dr. Will having been born in 1861 and Dr. Charlie in 1865. Pierre shared the brothers' dedication to excellence and continuous

Mother Alfred Moes founded Saint Marys Hospital, home to the surgical practice of Dr. William Worrall Mayo (center) and carried on by his sons, Drs. Charles Horace Mayo (left) and William James Mayo (right).

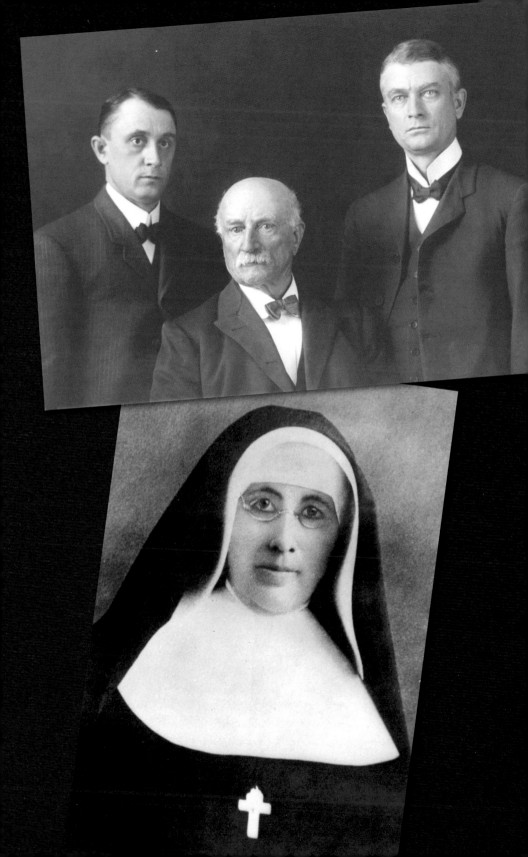

improvement, along with empathy for the poor and suffering. The Mayos considered themselves "moral custodians" of "the people's money" and calibrated their fees to the patient's ability to pay.

Dr. Will and Dr. Charlie practiced far from the urban centers of medicine, but they worked in an internationally recognized hospital, Saint Marys. The story of how that came to be must have warmed Pierre's heart.

On August 21, 1883, when Pierre was receiving treatment for his hearing condition as a boy in Luxembourg, Dr. Will was barely three months out of medical school and Charlie was the equivalent of a high school student. On that day a tornado devastated Rochester. W.W. Mayo was placed in charge of helping the injured survivors, assisted by his sons and other physicians in the community. They needed nurses and turned to Mother Alfred Moes, the founder of a religious community called the Sisters of St. Francis, who had opened a school in Rochester several years earlier.

For Pierre, it would have been providential that Mother Alfred was an immigrant from his homeland, Luxembourg, and bore the same last name as the pastor who was assigned to Berbourg about a year before Pierre left for America. She had been born in 1828 to a large, prosperous family in Remich, about 20 miles south of Berbourg.

Mother Alfred immediately sent several of her Franciscan Sisters, who were schoolteachers, to assist Dr. Mayo and his sons. When the crisis passed, she visited Dr. Mayo in his office and made an extraordinary offer: The Sisters would raise funds to construct a hospital and work there as nurses if he and his sons would take charge of the surgical care. Dr. Mayo resisted: It was an expensive, risky undertaking. Mother Alfred persisted: "With our faith and hope and energy," she assured him, "it will succeed."

And so it did. Saint Marys Hospital opened in 1889, when Pierre was taking his upper-level studies in Luxembourg. The hospital initially had capacity for 45 beds and quickly underwent one expansion after another. Rochester's remote location proved to be an advantage. The Mayo brothers and Franciscan Sisters were forced to rely upon one another and become self-sufficient.

With no medical hierarchy nearby, they were free to try bold new methods. As a result, Saint Marys was among the first hospitals in America to put the germ theory into practice. The railroad and early automobiles brought patients in great numbers from ever-widening distances. With an inherent sense of trust and teamwork, they welcomed partners and associates with complementary skills, creating the model of multispecialty integrated group practice.

By the time Pierre was in medical school and establishing his practice, the Mayos were publishing articles in national and international medical journals, reporting high volumes of complex surgical procedures with excellent results. This made Rochester just the place for Pierre to refer his patients, and for him to find the intellectual and professional stimulation he craved.

Pierre's boyhood experience as a patient who benefitted from a highly skilled, compassionate specialist likely informed his affiliation with the Mayo practice. Part of the high regard he earned from his own patients and other physicians stemmed from his openness to seek specialized opinions and refer his patients to other practitioners when the case required it. A.O. Mardorf, a Lutheran pastor who served in Titonka for nine years, wrote of Pierre:

> The people of the community also admired another quality of the good doctor. His diagnoses were always highly regarded by everyone. Furthermore, the doctor humbly knew his limitations, and therefore never once hesitated to send his patients on to hospital care or specialized treatment.

This outlook made Pierre a natural collaborator with the Mayos. We don't know exactly when the professional relationship began, but newspaper accounts linking Pierre and the Mayos started in the early 1900s and continued throughout his career. On November 1, 1907, a page-one story in the *Algona*

Courier reported:

> *Cecilia Grandjennet has been operated [on] by the*
> *Mayo Brothers at Rochester where she went on the*
> *advice of her local physician Dr. Sartor. The Mayos*
> *confirmed the diagnosis of Dr. Sartor in every detail.*
> *She will return tomorrow but will have to go back in*
> *3 months to have the operation completed.*

Pierre did more than refer patients to the Mayo brothers —
he also visited in person. Pierre signed the guest register of
Saint Marys Hospital on Monday, February 3, 1908.

What brought Pierre to Rochester that day isn't known, but
it must have been a pressing need to warrant leaving his patients and young family to travel during the Midwestern winter. He found himself in good company. About this time, the
medical journal *Canada Lancet* declared: "The rush of medical
visitors is unabated. . . . The little western town [is] slowly becoming the greatest post-graduate centre of the century, with
possibilities practically illimitable."

A doctor from St. Louis wrote:

> *Among the many physicians and surgeons who visit*
> *the Mayos are all kinds, from the most expert and*
> *renowned metropolitan surgeon to the plain country*
> *doctor who has brought in a case for operation. There*
> *were usually from twenty to thirty spectators every*
> *day.*

Physicians who signed the register on the same day as Pierre
included visiting surgeons from Virginia, North Dakota, Colo-
rado, Kansas, Ohio and Illinois; guests from abroad were included in other pages. Pierre fit comfortably into the mix. He
practiced in the country but had a cosmopolitan worldview.

So great was the crush of visitors that the Mayo brothers had
platforms made with wheels and handrails, so a group of ob-
servers could get close to the operating table with good visibil-
ity for all. As the hospital expanded, they had galleries for visitors built into the operating room, along with slanted mirrors
on the ceiling. Guests such as Pierre could look down into the
operating theater, ask questions and share information with

the surgical team, or look up at the ceiling for a detailed view of the procedure.

Wrote Helen Clapesattle, author of *The Doctors Mayo:*

> *There was as much to be heard as seen . . . for the brothers accompanied their operations with a running clinical commentary, reviewing the case history and the diagnosis, describing the conditions they found, and explaining what they did and why. In these talks they ranged through the whole of medical science, literature, and history, giving freely the convictions born of their wide reading and experience. . . .*

While many practitioners at the time jealously guarded their skills or charged fees to attend their operations, the Mayo brothers offered an open-door welcome, at no cost.

> *Both men were perfectly frank about their role, constantly telling visitors where they had picked up this good thing or that. . . . "I used to do this differently, but Moynihan showed me his method when he was here and it was better, so I use it now," Dr. Will would say. And Dr. Charlie, "The first time I tried this operation I got stuck at this point, but George Monk of Boston was here and he told me what to do."*

Pierre's collaboration with the Mayos coincided with the rise of specialization in the medical profession. The Mayo brothers began their careers as general surgeons, but over time Dr. Charlie developed expertise in operations of the head and neck while Dr. Will focused on abdominal surgery. This account in the Bancroft, Iowa, newspaper shows how Dr. Sartor, as a community-based practitioner, had clinical judgment that aligned with the specialty skills of the Mayos:

> *Dr. Sartor has the right to feel good, and he does. Mrs. J. M. McCowien for about a year has been ill. Many times Sartor said "Gall stones" and other great doctors said "No." Last week she went to Rochester and submitted to an operation, and if anyone wants to see a gall stone let them come to Sartor's office, where he will see one as large as an English*

walnut. Mrs. Mc is reported doing well. The stone is
certainly a wonder.

As other specialists joined the Mayo brothers, Pierre had more resources for the complex conditions he diagnosed among his patients.

For visiting physicians like Pierre, the social dimensions of trips to Rochester were equally important. Dr. Will and his wife, Hattie, as well as Dr. Charlie and his wife, Edith, had spacious homes and frequently hosted guests for meals or an overnight stay.

One can envision Pierre forming a bond with Dr. Charlie. They shared Chicago roots: Dr. Charlie graduated from Chicago Medical College, affiliated with Northwestern University, in 1888, eight years before Pierre graduated from Bennett Medical College. Dr. Charlie's wife, Edith, who was a nurse before their marriage, graduated from Woman's Hospital of Chicago in 1889. She shared her husband's interest in medicine and his warm sense of humor, which matched Pierre's. Dr. Charlie and Edith had a large, lively family with children about the age of Pierre and Mary's brood; several of the next generation of Mayo and Sartor children went into medicine. Dr. Charlie and Edith's son, Dr. Charles William (Chuck) Mayo, left this account of his "medically-saturated upbringing":

> *Almost every adult male in our family was a doctor*
> *and all their friends, it seemed, were doctors, and pla-*
> *toons of doctors constantly filled the guest rooms of*
> *our house. Dinner conversation rarely wavered from*
> *detailed shoptalk about the calamities that can befall*
> *the human interior, together with debate on their*
> *cause and cure.*

It is appealing to imagine Pierre as a guest in Dr. Charlie and Edith's dining room, contributing to the conversation on several levels. As a community-based physician, he could converse on par with specialists. In addition, Pierre's European background would have been of great interest to his Midwestern hosts. Dr. Will and Dr. Charlie not only welcomed visitors to Rochester. They also were known as the "Surgical Travelers of the World." Each year, the brothers took alternating trips abroad with a convivial group of relatives and colleagues. They toured hospitals and clinics, as well as museums, galleries and other cultural attractions. One can envision Pierre, with his knowledge of French and German, contributing to their appreciation of Europe.

Dr. Charlie and Pierre also shared an appreciation of rural life. In 1911, Dr. Charlie and Edith moved to a large country estate they called Mayowood. It eventually comprised about 3,000 acres, including several working farms. Dr. Charlie referred to himself as an agriculturist — a farmer, he said, made money working the land and spent it in town, while he earned his living as a surgeon in Rochester and spent it on his country pursuits. The sprawling house was Dr. Charlie's own design and he and Edith filled it with treasures from their travels around the world.

The Mayowood greenhouses would have been a special delight to Pierre. Growing up, his family in Luxembourg grew flowers as part of their farming enterprise; his brothers and in-laws developed thriving greenhouse businesses in Chicago. Dr. Charlie and Edith cultivated flowers on a grand scale: More than 60,000 chrysanthemum blooms drew thousands of visitors to the Mayowood annual show. The flowers were not all that riveted attention: "Visitors shown through the Mayowood greenhouses were always astonished when they came to an ell in which dark glass had been used to shut out the burning southern sunlight, for looking up they saw . . . [an] array of bones and body parts."

Dr. Charlie recycled plate glass X-rays from the Clinic to build his greenhouse!

There was another compelling reason why Pierre felt at home in Rochester. Mother Alfred Moes died before Pierre came to Rochester, but she left a rich legacy at Saint Marys Hospital, carried on by the Sisters of St. Francis — some of whom, like Mother Alfred and Pierre, came from Luxembourg, while others had French or German backgrounds. When he visited Saint Marys, Pierre would have witnessed a Catholic institution that upheld the highest professional standards in service to all — exactly the qualities of his personal ethos. Franciscan Sisters took an active role in every aspect of Saint Marys. Sister Joseph Dempsey, for example, was both the superintendent of the hospital and Dr. Will's first assistant in the operating room.

Even more remarkable was the spirit of cooperation. The Mayo brothers and many of their associates, most of them men, were humanistic Protestants. Yet they worked effectively and respectfully with devout Catholic Sisters who owned, managed and staffed Saint Marys Hospital — and they did so, bound not by a legal contract but by only a handshake between Dr. William Worrall Mayo and Mother Alfred Moes in 1883, which launched the whole endeavor.

To Pierre, this must have seemed the essence of why he came to the United States: He could express his faith while functioning in a pluralistic society; pursue intellectual rigor while living in a small town; and earn respect by focusing on service rather than money.

As his professional relationship with the Mayo brothers developed, there were an increasing number of reports in his hometown newspaper of Dr. Sartor's patients who went to Rochester. The chatty, neighborly way of conveying information through small-town news in the early 1900s had a role similar to social media today:

> *S.B. French . . . went to Rochester, Minn., last Sunday . . . He has not been feeling well lately and has lost a lot of flesh during the past few months. . . . Mrs. Jerry Heetland and little daughter Wanda [went] to Mayo Clinic. . . . The little Heetland babe has been having trouble with one of [her] feet.*

For physicians like Pierre who came to Rochester on professional visits, it was an exhilarating time. Two years before Pierre signed the guest book, a group of visiting physicians formed an informal discussion group called the International Surgeons Club (later shortened to Surgeons Club) to talk over what they learned from the Mayos and how to apply it. Yet for all they received, Pierre and his companions gave back in an important way.

The Mayo brothers' methods were so revolutionary that there was no effective description for how they worked. As their practice grew, its formal name — "The Doctors Mayo, Graham, Plummer and Judd" at one point — became ever more cumbersome. It was visiting physicians in the early 1900s who began to speak of going to "the Mayos' clinic."

The term "clinic" was used in Europe to describe a hospital-based teaching event and would have been instantly recognizable to a doctor from Luxembourg. We can imagine Pierre as an early, enthusiastic proponent of the title coined by his peers and soon picked up as a handy reference by the railroads, the popular press and, ultimately, by the designated institution itself.

As Dr. Will explained, the name "was not chosen by us but was given to us by our friends throughout the country, and as we became known by that name, it seemed expedient for us to adopt it eventually ourselves." One can say, therefore, that doctors like Pierre Sartor helped give the institution the name by which it is known today throughout the world — Mayo Clinic.

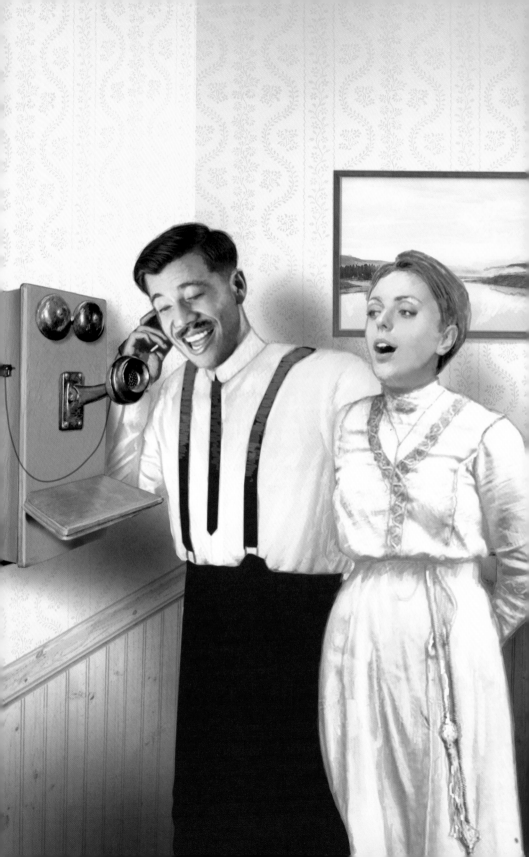

CHAPTER 11

Family Life

Bancroft, Iowa
1901-1918

LATE ONE EVENING, Pierre was finally home after seeing patients and catching up on work in his office. He was enjoying a glass of wine and leafing through a medical textbook. On sudden inspiration, he went to the wall-mounted telephone, cranked the handle and asked the operator to place a long-distance call to Chicago — to his father-in-law, Michael Winandy.

Such communications were unusual and expensive at the time, reserved for major life events. But Pierre's only purpose for this call was to have some fun. With Mr. Winandy on the line, Pierre burst into song in his distinctive accent flavored with French and German intonations, and the dialect of his native Luxembourg:

Oh, give me a home where the buffalo roam
And the deer and the antelope play. . . .

At some point, perhaps before "seldom is heard a discouraging

Pierre and Mary placed a long-distance telephone call, a rarity in the early 1900s, to serenade her family in Chicago and share their happiness at living in Iowa.

word," Mary chimed in, both of them sharing the moment with her father while also conveying in their choice of music and heartfelt rendition how much they enjoyed their Iowa "Home on the Range." Mr. Winandy's easy laugh conveyed his understanding and support.

The Winandys were a musical family, a trait that has continued across the generations. Pierre was an enthusiastic, albeit not an accomplished, vocalist, so for him and Mary to reach out in song, and for it to be received so enthusiastically by her father, is a demonstration of the warm regard that the families felt for each other.

This vignette in the Sartor family tradition also captures the spirit of confidence and well-being that many people felt in the era before the First World War. While by no means a positive time for everyone, Pierre and Mary would likely agree with historian Walter Lord, who wrote a book about the period entitled *The Good Years*. Pierre and Mary were established in Bancroft. He had a flourishing medical practice; she cultivated a garden in their spacious yard; and, for both of them, their growing family was a source of joy. If there is a theme for Pierre and Mary at this time, it would be the latticework pattern of communications and relationships as they cared for their children and coped with change. At times, they also opened their ample home to others. The 1910 census lists their household as including an 18-year-old boarder named Rosalie whose occupation was "teacher, rural school."

Pierre and Mary were blessed with six children: Mary (May), who was born in High Ridge in 1899 and accompanied them on the train trip to Iowa; Magdalene, born in 1902; Guido, born in 1906; Mercedes, born in 1908; Alice, born in 1912; and Anthony, born in 1914.

During these years, Mary realized that an occasional telephone call home would not suffice. She had grown up in a large family and had been, in many respects, a surrogate mother to her younger siblings. Mary missed them and they, in turn, clamored to see her and her children.

Thus began a pattern, extended over several years and duly

reported in the local paper, whereby Mary left Iowa in the summer, taking the children for a six-week visit to Chicago. It speaks to the strength of their marriage that at a time of traditional norms, she could express her wishes for such a trip, journeying without her husband, and Pierre would agree. After all, Pierre had left Mary, at a much more tender age, before their marriage, to explore Iowa for months at a time, and he understood the fairness of her request.

The telephone — a rarity in private homes — became their point of connection. They spoke during her summer absences so Pierre could hear the children, whether a baby's coo, a toddler's patter or an older child's report on his or her activities. Pierre and Mary exchanged postcards and confirmed the date for her return. He met her at the train station for a joyous reunion.

Each year, Mary returned home with a sophisticated air, rice powder lightly puffed onto her face, lips with a bit of gloss, her hair styled with pomade. Pierre greeted his wife with a scent of cloves and soap — and not the antiseptic kind.

Each year, Mary returned home in August. For several years, nine months later, she delievered another child. By the time Guido was 12 years old, he asked his mother, with a display of the precocious forthrightness that would later serve him well as a pediatrician: *Why are the babies almost always born in May?* Indeed, of the Sartors' six children, all five who were born in Iowa, Guido included, had birthdays that month.

Mary Magdalene, her refined Victorian upbringing tempered by years on the prairie, explained: *After my summer away, Pa is so happy to see me. . . .*

One year, Pierre accompanied Mary to Chicago, but the occasion was not a happy one. Mrs. Winandy, Mary's chronically frail mother, died before reaching her 50th birthday. That Pierre would make the trip was a sign of his respect for Mary's family. But even then, he was gone barely two days. *I am needed*, Pierre said, referring to his patients and explaining his prompt return to Bancroft. In Minnesota, the Mayo brothers alternated between staying at home to mind the practice and venturing out to see other medical centers. As a physician in solo practice, Pierre remained at home with the stated reason of being near his patients.

Pierre kept in touch with his brothers and their families, but a review of newspaper social columns over the decades indicates that most visits took place when the elder Sartors headed west, such as a trip that Ferdinand and Margaretha made to the Black Hills with a stop in Iowa, rather than Pierre going back to Chicago. Multiple reasons were likely involved. There is no question that Pierre was devoted to his patients, which limited his travels. But he had also spent formative periods of his life away from his family — when he received treatment for his hearing condition, followed by years of education. From early adolescence, he was a visitor in his family's home. Then he immigrated to the United States and, within a short time, moved away from his brothers and his wife's family. All things considered, Pierre was comfortable on his own.

These and other factors came to the fore when Pierre had an opportunity to visit Luxembourg but did not. In the decade he had been in America, Pierre maintained periodic contact with his relatives in Berbourg. One evening in 1904, Pierre was on a telephone call from a patient. Mary was darning socks. There came a knock on the door. It was a telegram for Pierre, edged in black, from his older sister Liss in Berbourg. Their father, Mathias, was dead. The news was brutal: He froze to death in a blizzard while walking home from a funeral.

Mathias had launched Pierre on his career and, ultimately, on the path his life would take. *First things first*, Mathias had said, arranging treatment for Pierre's hearing problem and then for an education far surpassing what others in the family could possibly hope for; but when Mathias needed Pierre most, his son the doctor was not there.

Will you go home? Mary asked.

Pierre could almost hear his sister Liss: *Pittchen? Will you come home?*

But Pierre knew the answer. Within a breath, he replied to Mary, but in his heart, he spoke also to his family across the ocean: *I cannot. My patients are here.*

During these years, Pierre and Mary also faced medical needs within their family. Their youngest child, Anthony, was frail. A pattern emerged, spanning the generations. Pierre had been a frail boy, youngest of his brothers, not allowed to roughhouse and tumble, and the family called him Pittchen. Anthony, who also had health problems, was the baby of their family; for his fair coloring and gentle ways, his family called him Tinnie.

And just as Ferdinand had devoted himself to Pierre, Guido, the sturdy older brother of this generation, became caretaker and confidant to Anthony. This experience, in turn, helped shape Guido's life and career.

Pierre struggled for years to find the cause of and cure for Anthony's poor health, which must have called forth memories. His own doctor in Luxembourg had solved his chronic ear problem at a time when successful treatment was far from certain. Three decades later, couldn't Pierre do the same for his own son? With his stethoscope he could examine the boy. But there was no treatment available for Anthony's weak heart.

Pierre and Mary's growing concern for Anthony marks the end of this period. On the horizon were crises of national and global magnitude: the First World War and the influenza pandemic.

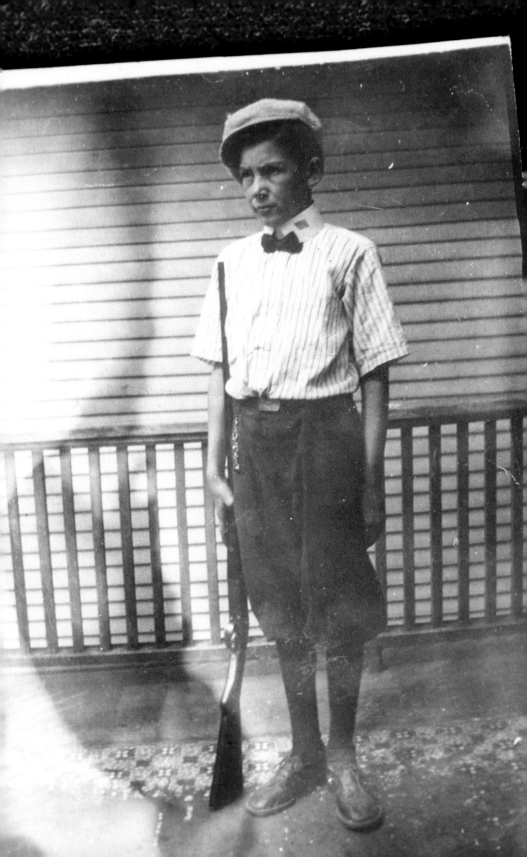

CHAPTER 12

The Great War Comes Home to Small-Town America

Bancroft, Iowa
1914-1918

FROM THE CROWNED HEADS OF EUROPE to the farmers of Kossuth County, Iowa, no one could have predicted the cataclysm that occurred in the summer of 1914. The assassination of Franz Ferdinand, heir to the throne of the Austro-Hungarian Empire, and his wife, in Sarajevo, Bosnia, on June 28 unleashed a cascade of events that engulfed much of the globe in unprecedented conflict, known then as the Great War and later as the First World War.

Today it is difficult to imagine the upheaval that the conflict brought. Europe had been free of continent-wide strife since the Napoleonic era nearly a century before. In the United States, the Civil War was some 50 years in the past. The 19th and early 20th centuries had seen times of conflict, but families like the Sartors, Winandys and Mayos could cross international borders with ease. Commerce and culture flowed smoothly among countries.

At age 11, Pierre and Mary's eldest son, Guido, joined the Rifle Club in the patriotic spirit of World War I.

Pierre, Mary and the Mayo brothers all had immigrant roots, being newcomers or one generation removed. They considered themselves patriotic Americans and, in outlook, something akin to citizens of the world. In the spring of 1914, Dr. Will Mayo made one of his annual trips abroad. He praised the cosmopolitan spirit of medicine: ". . . science has no country." A few weeks later, Europe was at war — an industrialized conflict that involved millions of combatants, destroying cities and landscapes.

For Pierre and Mary, the sudden coming of war to the heart of Europe was a wrenching experience. Luxembourg, their homeland, is located between France and Germany. Pierre and Mary valued the cultures of both countries, now locked in deadly conflict with each other.

The neutrality of Luxembourg had been guaranteed for decades by international law — as had that of nearby Belgium, whose treaty protection one German official dismissed as "a scrap of paper." Luxembourg lay directly in the path of Germany's plan to invade France.

In one of the gallant stories of that time, Marie-Adélaïde, the Grand Duchess of Luxembourg and its reigning monarch, protested the German invasion. At 20 years of age, she was beautiful, devoutly Catholic and much given to the wearing of pearls. The Grand Duchess made a striking figure, but her remonstrance was to no avail. German troops surged into Luxembourg, which was occupied from August 2, 1914, until the war ended on November 11, 1918. For Pierre's and Mary's families and others who lived there, it was a time of extreme duress.

At war's start, the United States was resolutely neutral; the Iowa prairie was far removed from Flanders Fields in Western Europe, where the conflict raged. But the war had steep costs, not just for the men in the trenches, but for every life and heart.

Pierre was torn. According to letters he received, many of his relatives in Luxembourg were still warm to Germany and tolerated the military occupation, despite shortages of food and other staples. A relative praised the German soldiers. A friend wrote of waiting for her German fiancé, an air force pilot, to return.

From his years in the United States, Pierre had developed a broader perspective. After the German invasion of Belgium, Luxembourg and France, Pierre saw Germany as the aggressor. This was a source of distress, given the strong German roots of people in Bancroft. Pierre and Mary could feel public opinion turn in the face of German atrocities, which were condemned in the press as the "rape of Belgium." Public outrage intensified after a German submarine sank the British ocean liner *Lusitania* on May 7, 1915, with the loss of nearly 1,200 civilian passengers and crew. One of the casualties was Evan Jones, age 65, from Ottumwa, Iowa, about 230 miles southeast of Bancroft.

The United States entered the war on the side of the Allies — led by England and France — against Germany in April 1917. Patriotic posters urged Americans to "Do Your Bit," and Pierre was eager to contribute. That summer, Pierre applied for a commission in the Medical Reserve Corps of the U.S. Army. One of the 32 questions on the form was "What opportunities for instruction or practice of operative surgery have you had?" It is perhaps a reflection of Pierre's experience with Tonsil Tuesdays and his affiliations with local hospitals and Mayo Clinic that he replied, "Active practice."

The form he filled out — and the rejection letter he received — are in the lockbox.

Pierre was 46 years old, but it still hurt to be turned down by the military. He was an American citizen and loved his adopted country. All the while, doctors around him were entering the armed forces. The Mayo brothers worked with the U.S. Surgeon General, coordinating medical services for the military. Mary's brothers, Michael and Peter, were in uniform.

As time passed, Pierre realized his greatest service would be to his patients. As more men and women entered the military and related services, those on the home front — spouses, youth, the elderly — faced daunting challenges to provision the war effort and meet civilian needs as well.

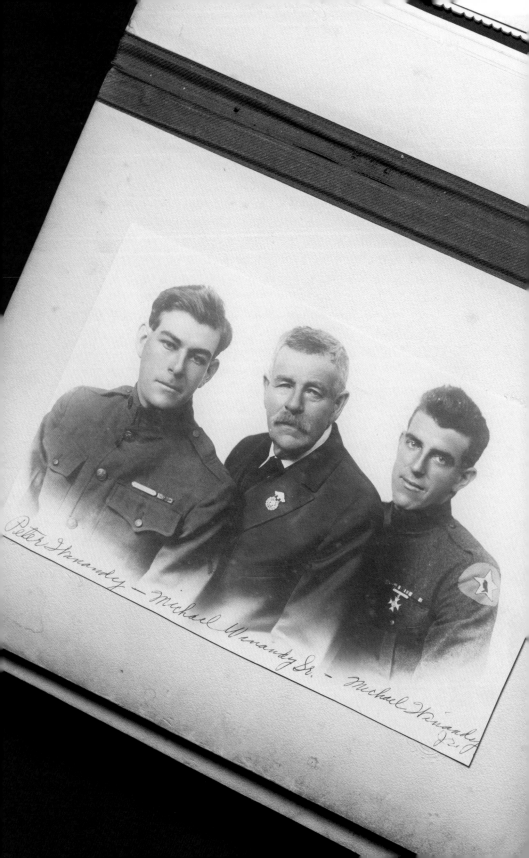

Peter Hernandy — Michael Wernandy Sr. — Michael Hernandy Jr.

Mary prayed every day that the war would end, but the conflict raged on.

Mary and her friends were reading and discussing a book entitled *Over the Top* by Arthur Guy Empey, which was being serialized in the local newspaper. It provided a vivid first-person account of combat conditions. *Over the Top* included this plaintive song, heard in the trenches of France:

> *I want to go home. I want to go home.*
> *I don't want to go to the trenches no more.*
> *. . . Take me over the sea, where the Allemand can't get*
>   *at me.*
> *Oh my! I don't want to die! I want to go home.*

All over Bancroft were women with frightened eyes, worried for their sweethearts, husbands, brothers and sons. Soon there were women with drawn, brittle faces, having lost menfolk in the war.

Mothers keep agoing on, said Pierre.

For her part, Mary devoted her knitting skills to the Red Cross, redoubling her effort to produce items that could be used by those in need at home and soldiers and war refugees overseas — socks and sweaters, bibs and other garments.

But the war seemed to invade every corner of their lives. On Mary's dining room table landed a hog census notice. It leaned against a china plate, like a place card for a formal luncheon or dinner. One of Pierre and Mary's children received the card at school, along with instructions to bring it home. The government was conducting a census of hogs in the state of Iowa. Officials wanted to know how much pork could be depended on for home consumption and how much could be exported to America's soldiers and allies.

The Sartors were not livestock farmers, so this survey did not apply to them. But the regulations and recommendations

Two of Mary's brothers, Peter (left) and Michael Jr. (right), wore their military uniforms in this portrait with their father, Michael Sr. Another brother, Alfred, also served in World War I.

continued.

A second card described the sugar shortage. It recommended fruit syrups, honey, maple sugar, sorghum or molasses, all to reduce consumption of granulated sugar. Mary noted on her recipe cards: "Honey with a little salt for jam and marmalade. Let stand for five or six days before using." The salt taste would disappear. "Three-four cups sugar substitute to 1-2 tablespoon salt per pound of fruit."

More and more farm goods appeared on Pierre's front porch as payment for his services, always with a note. Farmers had sick children but no money.

Pierre was paid in crops and livestock . . . then, again, sometimes not. Pierre had the gift of finding humor, even under duress. As he recalled: *Once a farmer said he was going to slaughter a cow, and he would pay me with half of it. Except the farmer changed his mind. "I'm sorry, Doc, but the cow got well."*

The war pinched their world, it seemed, on all fronts.

Pierre and Mary's eldest son, Guido, on the cusp of adolescence, once asked his father: *Are we poor?*

Yes, we are, Pierre said. They were as well off as people on farms, though, he reminded Guido. *We all have food, at least.*

Are farmers poor, too?

Poorer than us.

Pierre had just one more thing to say, and it went into his papers: "Nothing easy."

As war engulfed Europe, Mary, standing, continued her visits to Chicago. The Sartor children are May (far right) and Magdalene (second from right). Seated are Mercedes (second from left) and Guido (third from left). Mary's sister is seated, with her children filling in the picture.

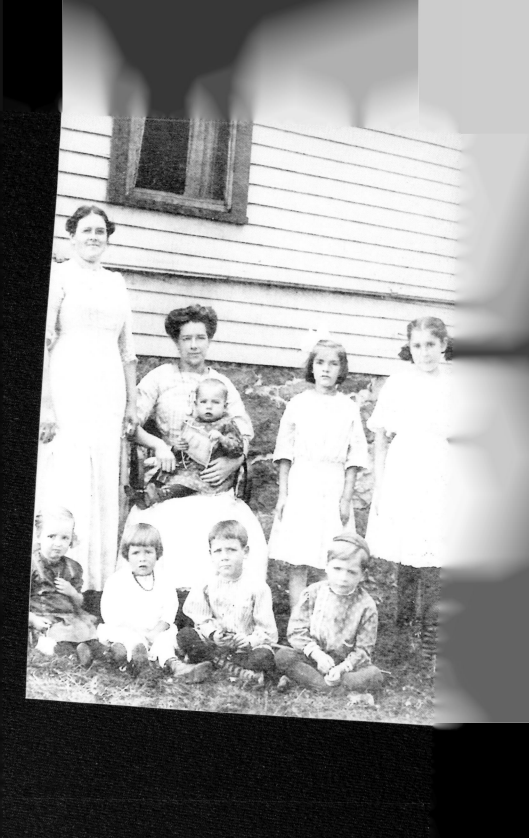

um seufze ich mit Herzensinbrunst zu
Dir und rufe mit allen Kräften meiner
Seele zu Dir auf: O Jesu, Du Sohn
Gottes, erbarme Dich meiner! O Jesu,
Du Sohn Maria, erbarme Dich meiner!
Dich meiner, Du Jesu, Du Sohn Davids, erbarme
Dich meiner, jetzt und in der Stunde
meines Todes! Amen.

Litanei vom allerheiligsten Namen Jesu.

Herr, erbarme Dich unser!
Christe, erbarme Dich unser!
Herr, erbarme Dich unser!
Jesu, höre uns!
Jesu, erhöre uns!
Gott Vater vom Himmel —
Gott Sohn, Erlöser der Welt,
Gott heiliger Geist, ein einiger
Heilige Dreifaltigkeit,

} Erbarme Dich unser!

Sohn des lebendigen
lanz des Vaters,
des ewigen Lichtes,
der Glorie,
der Gerechtigkeit,

} Dich unser!

Jesu, Du Sohn der Jungfrau Maria,
Du liebenswürdiger Jesu,
Du wunderbarer Jesu,
Jesu, Du starker Gott,
Jesu, Du Vater der Ewigkeit,
Jesu, Du Engel des großen Rath-
schlusses,
Du mächtigster Jesu,
Du geduldigster Jesu,
Du gehorsamster Jesu,
Jesu, sanft und demüthig von Herzen,
Jesu, Du Freund der Keuschheit,
Jesu, Du unser Freund,
Jesu, Du Gott des Friedens,
Jesu, Du Urheber des Lebens,
Jesu, Du Vorbild der Tugenden,
Jesu, Du Eiferer der Seelen,
Jesu, unser Gott,
Jesu, unsere Zuflucht,
Jesu, Du Vater der Armen,
Jesu, Du Schatz der Gläubigen,
Jesu, Du guter Hirt,
Jesu, Du wahres Licht,
Jesu, Du ewige Weisheit,
Jesu, Du unendliche Güte,
Jesu, unser Weg und Leben,
Jesu, Du Freude der Engel,

} Erbarme Dich unser!

CHAPTER 13

Time to Move?

Bancroft, Iowa
Winter and Spring 1918

PIERRE HAD BEEN TURNED DOWN by the military. But a confluence of personal and professional factors, and the gathering storm of what became the influenza pandemic, would put him on the front lines, right at home.

It began innocently enough with a question of just where his home would be.

About 12 miles southeast from Bancroft, Dr. Robert M. Wallace announced he was leaving the little town of Titonka, Iowa, where he practiced, to move to Algona, the seat of Kossuth County. Dr. Wallace wanted closer access to the hospital facilities in Algona.

Dr. Wallace and Dr. Sartor were longtime friends. Both had graduated from Bennett Medical College, and both had applied to join the Kossuth County Medical Society at the same meeting in 1908. So, it was not a surprise when Dr. Wallace

Pierre enjoyed reading devotional books. The pages shown here, written in German, are from Mary's First Communion book and speak to Pierre and Mary's faith.

contacted Pierre to ask if he would leave Bancroft and take over the Titonka practice. Pierre was needed there, even more than in Bancroft. At that time, two other doctors worked in Bancroft; Dr. Wallace's departure would leave Titonka without a physician. Dr. Wallace's offer of Titonka granted Pierre the chance to be the sole medical provider for the community.

It was a flattering invitation. But was Pierre's family ready to leave their hometown? Much had changed since he and Mary had settled in Bancroft 17 years before. Pierre's practice and the family were flourishing. Their daughters, May, Magdalene, Mercedes and Alice, according to the norms of the time, were busy learning the skills to manage a home in anticipation of getting married and having families of their own. Active in the Girl Scouts, they were at or approaching the age of attending cakewalks, box lunches and barn dances, events to be savored with lifelong girlfriends and newfound beaux in Bancroft.

And the boys? Here, Pierre took stock. They both were intelligent and good-hearted. But Anthony was frail. Clearly, he would need help all his life. His heart condition showed no sign of improvement.

By contrast, Guido, the older son, was robust. But he was also a handful. Pierre was not easily provoked, but in extremity he would issue an oath in French, German, English or the dialect of Luxembourg that translates roughly as *A million thousand thunders!* His elder son, Americanized and worldly by early adolescence, would reply good-naturedly, *That's some swearing. . . .*

In the summer of 1917, his parents decided that Guido should accompany Mary on her summer visit to Chicago. Guido needed a change of scene. And Pierre loved the fact that Guido would spend time with his relatives, including his grandfather, Michael Winandy. The boy had been eight when he had visited last, in the summer of 1914, when the war began in Europe. This time Guido could show off the drills he learned in the local Rifle Club. He impressed his grandfather and Uncle Alfred ("Freddie"), who as a child had brought Pierre and Mary together in their courting days. "Guido put some pop in it!" Grandpa Winandy wrote in a postcard to Pierre.

Guido thrived during this visit. He loved the abundance and variety of flowers under glass in the Winandy greenhouses. Guido became a little Luxie, developing increased pride in his heritage over that summer. How his grandfather laughed; Mr. Winandy was so pleased. And that news delighted Pierre. The summer in Chicago fed Guido's high spirits.

Guido was going on 12. Back home in Bancroft, he cut cords of wood for Pierre's office, stacked wood for the kitchen fire and hauled coal to the house. In addition, he had a real job that put him under other people's authority, a good experience for the lad. Opposite their home was the Swedish Lutheran Church, which employed Guido to ring the bells. Pierre was proud of Guido.

But, one day word reached Pierre: His son was seen in the belfry of the church, legs dangling out the opening, drinking a soda, waving to friends. Pierre was livid.

But, Pa, said Guido, oblivious to his father's reaction. *I can watch the baseball game from up there!*

He didn't do it again. But it was clear Guido needed a more demanding job. And Guido had learned a lesson: Stay focused while working. Perhaps father and son both needed more of a challenge.

But a move?

More was at stake than Pierre realized at the time.

There is strong evidence that in the first weeks of 1918, just as Pierre was contemplating the move to Titonka, a new influenza virus — which became the global pandemic — came into being in Haskell County, Kansas. Its exact cause is unknown. But the pattern of migratory birds and the presence of large numbers of livestock could support development of a virus that spread to humans and began to mutate with severe, and deadly, results.

Located about 660 miles southwest of Kossuth County, Iowa, what one might call Ground Zero of the 1918 influenza pandemic had notable connections to Pierre's story. It was a western prairie setting, the environment that so attracted

Pierre. The "flu" first appeared on farms and ranches and in small towns, the types of places where Pierre most enjoyed working. And it was first documented by a physician like Pierre. Dr. Loring Miner had a scientific education and classical tastes, yet he thrived on the frontier. He practiced solo and earned the devotion of his patients.

From late January through mid-March 1918, outbreaks of influenza consumed Dr. Miner's attention and energy. The condition itself, and the timing of its outbreak, were not new — influenza in one form or another was typical at that time of year. But there were key differences: Dr. Miner saw cases that spread rapidly, causing unusually severe symptoms and, far too often, death. And while influenza typically threatened children and the elderly, pregnant women and the infirm, this form of the disease struck otherwise healthy, vigorous young adults. With his perspective based in the classics, Dr. Miner would have naturally drawn comparisons to the plague of Athens in ancient times.

As this dangerous form of influenza swirled in Haskell County, Kansas, Pierre and Mary faced an immediate and deeply personal question. In any discussion of whether they should move to Titonka, one issue was inescapable: The nearest Catholic church of significance was in the nearby town of Wesley. In Titonka, there were few Catholics and few, if any, immigrants from Luxembourg.

Faith and ethnicity were core elements of Pierre's and Mary's lives. The last words his father spoke to him before Pierre boarded ship for America admonished fidelity to the Catholic Church. Pierre and Mary shared roots in Luxembourg and, when leaving Chicago for Bancroft, made sure those elements were present in their life in Iowa. Indeed, those elements were thriving: Less than three years before, their adopted St. John the Baptist Church in Bancroft, many of whose parishioners were immigrants or the children of immigrants from Luxembourg, had dedicated a beautiful new structure.

What about Mary? As a young married woman with a babe in arms, she had left the comforts and cultural attainments of her family's home in Chicago. Now, middle-aged and the mother of six children, she faced another move to a smaller, more remote location. Her thoughts at this juncture are unknown, but her actions demonstrate full support.

However long the deliberations took, there came a time when events drove the decision. Pierre learned that Dr. Wallace would not be moving to Algona, after all — Dr. Wallace was drafted and making plans to enter the military.

Pierre heard a call of his own, as clear as when a bugler sounded reveille. It was the mantra that guided Pierre throughout his adult life — to go where "I am needed." He would make the move.

To ease his own and his family's transition to their new home in Titonka, Pierre purchased a book of prayers for devotions at home when they could not travel to Wesley for Sunday Mass. More than a century later, this prayer book is a cherished heirloom in the Sartor family. Its pages are frayed and creased at the edges — many of them turned dark from oil on the fingers that held the book tight — evidence of repeated, fervent use.

Pierre would open this prayer book on many occasions in the challenging times ahead.

Minnesota

LAKOTA •

BUFFALO Center

Bancroft •

Winnebago County

Slough

Titonka

•Woden

• BURT

Lake George

Crystal Lake

WESLEY

Britt •

Eagle Lake

Algona •

Kossuth County

Hancock County

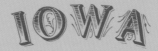

IOWA

CHAPTER 14

"My Titonka"

Titonka, Iowa
Spring and Summer 1918

PIERRE AND HIS FAMILY settled comfortably into their new life in Titonka.

Their house at 411 Main Street North is still standing: a two-story, wood frame residence. You enter the front by climbing a flight of steps to the screened-in porch. Go through the porch and the front door opens to a combined living-dining area — an early concept of the "great room" design — with a bay window in the dining area. I have many memories of being there as a child and young adult. I visited again in the early 2000s after family members at last sold it and the new owners used it as a teahouse called the Sartor House. Today the residence is in private hands.

Titonka had been incorporated in 1898 following railroad construction in that part of Kossuth County. By the time of the 1910 census, its population was 278, which would increase to 418 in 1920; of significance to Pierre, while few residents were

This map shows the location of activities associated with Pierre and Mary's family in the World War I era.

from Luxembourg, many people in Titonka spoke German. Like Bancroft, the community of Titonka served more than its immediate residents. Titonka also was a gathering place for people from nearby farms and hamlets who could reach the town by horseback or buggy over trails and rough, unpaved roads.

Pierre's fascination with the West found resonance in the town's name. Titonka derives from the Sioux language: "ta" for "large" and "tanka" for "black." To the Sioux, the concept of "large black" described the bison. This term and the importance of bison to the Sioux culture are highlighted in the film *Dances with Wolves*.

Pierre established his practice on Main Street, a convenient walk from home. The space Pierre leased for his medical duties included a small entry and waiting room as well as an adjoining office and examination room with a fireplace for heat. Before Dr. Wallace's deployment, he and Pierre spent a week together visiting patients. Between the cordial introduction from Dr. Wallace and Pierre's winning personality, townspeople and rural folk responded with a hearty welcome for their new doctor.

But Pierre being Pierre, it was inevitable that his move to a new community would include a sartorial statement — with predictable results.

Pierre repeated his experience from when he moved to Bancroft in 1901. On his first Sunday in Titonka, Pierre saw fit to stroll about wearing his Prince Albert suit with top hat and cane. He followed his constitutional by attending Mass in the nearby town of Wesley. If Pierre had been promenading on Michigan Avenue, the fashionable thoroughfare in Chicago, passersby would have stared at his outfit, which now was a quarter-century out of date. Among the denim- and gingham-clad farm folk who were his new neighbors and patients, one can imagine the response.

I thought a man of my station should wear such. And so, I wore the suit to Wesley to Mass, Pierre recounted years later in a tape-recorded interview. *But I heard laughter behind me. The mayor wore none such; no one else did. I did not do that again.*

Significantly, however, this was the last time Pierre felt the need to assert his status. As a boy, a young man and an early career professional, Pierre had aspired to social standing — even as he embraced a life of medical service rather than financial gain. Now, it seems, that tension was finally resolved. Over the next 40 years, he would wear this distinctive outfit again on ceremonial occasions with a nod to history, but not to claim status for himself. In a real sense, when Pierre packed up his formal attire after this initial and chuckle-inspiring venture upon moving to Titonka, he had come home. At last, Dr. Sartor was where he was meant to be.

For his family, the move also seems to have been a positive change. The only account of friction that survives in family lore recalls the time when Guido, the new kid in town, came running home, all flustered. On his trail in close pursuit was an older boy who bullied him from the sidewalk, shouting: *There are guns in the vestibule of your church! Catholics got guns in Wesley!* This boy had chased Guido home, right up his own steps!

Pierre waved his son's tormentor on. It was hard for Pierre to comprehend.

At times like this, Pierre turned to his long view of life. He did not tolerate prejudice, probably because the people of Luxembourg, even with the strains that are inherent in any society, understood the importance of getting along with the countries and cultures that were their close neighbors.

But on that day, Pierre's religion was challenged. He closed the front door. A ruckus over guns? No, not about guns. He knew there were no guns in their church. Guido's acquaintance had small vision, Pierre said, and he would not allow Guido to return the ill will of the bully's anti-Catholic prejudice. Subject closed. Pierre's message to Guido: *A prayer by a good person of any religion is good.*

Pierre's respect for other points of view would serve him well as the new doctor in a community of mixed faiths and ethnicities.

Guido had a far more positive experience when Pierre made an announcement to the family: It was time to purchase an auto-

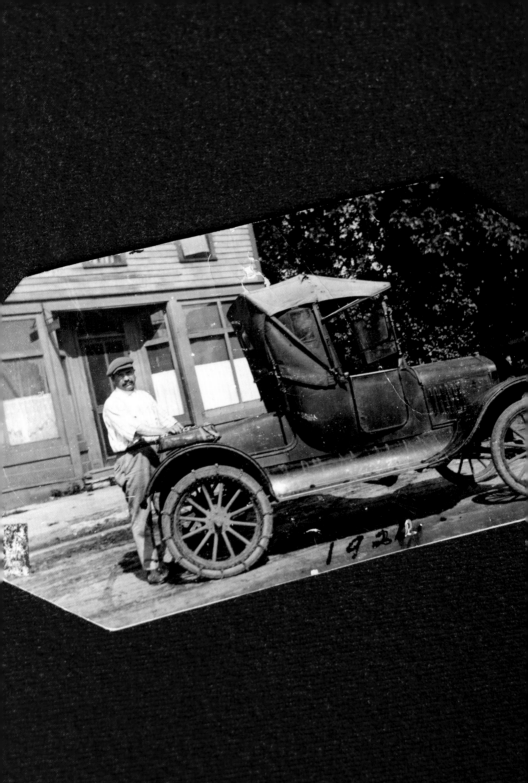

mobile. He needed it to reach his widely dispersed patients.

Automobiles had been available since the turn of the century. In 1901, the *Journal of the American Medical Association* published a report by Dr. Charlie Mayo that was intended to help physicians choose between models powered by gasoline, electricity and steam. His conclusion: "Automobiles at present are more or less of a pleasure vehicle for good roads, their perfection not being such as to warrant the physician who purchases one in selling his horse."

By now, however, automobiles were a fixture in cities like Chicago and Des Moines; there were even some on the streets of Bancroft and a few in Titonka. For Pierre, getting a car was a major change in his life and medical practice. Of course, having a car was no guarantee of easy mobility on primitive roads. In the flu-burdened winter to come and for several years afterward, heavy rains and snow would force Pierre to use a horse cart or sleigh.

But Pierre was determined to have a car, and he ensured the vehicle would be as useful as possible. It was not a luxury model but, rather, a Ford: mass-produced, simple to run and repair, the type of car that was reshaping transportation and many other facets of American life. Pierre noted with approval that the windshield offered protection from bugs, rain and snow.

For Guido, getting the car was a highlight of his life. He lived to age 98 and always remembered that day, coming six days after his 12th birthday. Throughout his life, Guido was enthralled with automobiles. Decades later, he wrote down a set of memories for his grandchildren. In reply to "What was the first present you remember receiving?" he answered, "A car run by foot pedals." Now his family was getting a real car.

Even more memorable: On that day he also crossed paths with the love of his life . . . although it took several years for them both to figure that out.

Pierre's Model T Ford, nicknamed the "Riggedy-Jig," had a central role in many family adventures.

There was another family shopping for a car that day. Henry and Wilhelmina Recker were making a purchase as well, and they brought along their daughter Luella. The families knew each other; Guido and Luella attended school together for a few years when living in Bancroft, and Pierre had delivered Luella's sister, Leone. Since then, just as the Sartors had relocated to Titonka, the Reckers had moved to a farm near Buffalo Center, Iowa.

We don't know if Guido and Luella exchanged stolen glances in the car dealership, but it is a fact they would be married and have a long, happy life together; I am the second of their four children. It is a favorite story in the Sartor family that, just as Pierre and Mary unknowingly shared a trolley ride to the World's Fair years before they met, a generation later, their son Guido was in a car shop with his future wife, Luella, when they were youngsters.

If Guido had romance on his mind that day, it would have been focused on the lure of the open road. It is a sign of Guido's natural mechanical ability — and the loose regulations of the time — that Pierre let his son drive the new car home.

In the book for his grandchildren, Guido proudly wrote that he "learned [to drive] at 12 years." He and the car became inseparable.

Guido's automotive adventures were just starting. Later that summer, he embarked upon a much longer trip, which involved driving his mother about 400 miles to Chicago. After years of taking the train to visit her family, Mary made her first extended journey by car. Pierre saw them off. *Twelve miles an hour in towns!* Pierre admonished his son, who had already earned the nickname "Swifty Sartor" for his lifelong practice of arriving barely in the nick of time for any appointment. The parental warning continued: *Over that and you will get fined!*

Guido traversed the Midwest's nascent interstate road system. A loose, community-based consortium of "Good Roads" committees helped link destinations together via gravel-covered and, occasionally, paved surfaces. The Mayo brothers were leaders of the "Good Roads" effort in Rochester, Minnesota, to provide access for farmers who wanted to come to town and patients who were traveling in record numbers to Mayo Clinic. Highways and the numbering system as we know them were years in the future, so Guido navigated by the "red ball" route, looking for telephone and telegraph poles that were painted with a white band and red ball in the center. Of course, roadside lights, service stations and amenities such as motels and restaurants were nonexistent.

It is pleasant to imagine young Guido gallantly chauffeuring his mother on the prairie roads. They likely wore goggles and linen "dusters," the approved attire of "automobilists" at the time, and had luggage strapped to the running boards of their car. Pilot and passenger arrived at High Ridge in good order, and their kinfolk gave them a warm welcome.

But there was a tinge of anxiety in the summer of 1918. The war and influenza were coming home to the Sartor family.

The letters and other news accounts that Pierre received from Europe were irregular, given the predatory destroyers and submarines that sank ships on the open sea. We do not know when Pierre learned of the murder that summer of former Tsar Nicholas II of Russia and his wife, the Empress Alexandra, and their five children, as well as several members of their household staff. Nicholas had abdicated his throne the year before, and his family had endured increasing hardship as the Bolshevik Revolution engulfed Russia. Throughout his life, Pierre told stories about his ocean voyage to America, during which he met an anarchist who wanted to kill the tsar, so the death of Nicholas II and his family must have registered with Pierre. Although their lives were quite different, Pierre and Mary were contemporaries of Nicholas and Alexandra; both couples had large families with adolescent children, most of whom were daughters, and each family had a youngest son who was sickly: Alexis Romanov had hemophilia while Anthony Sartor had congenital heart disease.

The timing of Pierre's professional transition is significant. While he was establishing his practice in Titonka, the influenza virus that circulated in sparsely populated Haskell County,

189

Kansas, found its way to Camp Funston, part of the massive Fort Riley military installation in the north-central part of the state. There, thousands of men were packed together in quarters that were hastily built and inadequately supplied. On March 4, a base camp cook reported symptoms of influenza. Within hours, dozens more men were stricken and within three weeks, more than 1,100 soldiers were hospitalized, while countless others sought care for milder symptoms at Fort Riley's satellite infirmaries. The constant coming-and-going that is part of life at a military encampment — troops mustering in, taking leave and deploying elsewhere, visitors arriving, suppliers making deliveries — ensured rapid, widespread transmission of the virus to other military centers and communities in the United States and abroad.

In its issue for April 5, 1918, *Public Health Reports*, a weekly journal of the U.S. Public Health Service, carried a notice from Dr. Miner regarding "influenza of severe type" in Haskell County. This in itself would have been noteworthy since influenza was so common that physicians were not required to report it and no state or federal health agency tracked it. For *Public Health Reports* to carry a warning about influenza meant something quite different was taking place. Other medical journals also published articles about influenza that season.

In the weeks and months that followed, the condition became known as Spanish flu, which is a misnomer. Under wartime censorship, Allied governments suppressed news of the outbreak among their military forces. Spain was neutral in the Great War and its relatively free press covered the spread of influenza, especially when it struck King Alfonso XIII in late May. As a nickname, "Spanish flu" gave an identity to the mysterious, potentially fatal condition and helped focus public attention, despite the inaccurate description of its origin. Spaniards, for their part, referred to the disease as the "French flu."

Along with perusing medical literature, doctors read about severe cases of influenza in the popular press. Pierre never missed the *Des Moines Register*. He and his colleagues discussed articles from the paper at monthly meetings of the Kossuth County Medical Society. Important medical news that might need immediate attention was shared by telephone, with doctors who volunteered to work the "telephone tree," calling colleagues on a prearranged list. News on the telephone wire could travel quickly across the county and throughout the state, just as branches bring moisture to the tiniest of leaves.

It was a telephone call to the Sartor residence that brought Pierre his first case of influenza. The patient was in Chicago. It was his brother-in-law Alfred, the same Freddie who introduced Pierre and Mary with such poise in their courting days, and who had cheered for Guido as he demonstrated his Rifle Club drill.

Pierre remembered that night for the rest of his life. He was in bed, exhausted, frustrated that he had not been able to get to as many patients as he had wanted to — needed to — that day. In the bedroom doorway stood Mary, who had taken the call. *Freddie is in dire straits*, she said.

Up in an instant, Pierre went to the telephone, mounted on a wall near the front door. He listened to Alfred and did his best to diagnose and prescribe treatment by long distance.

There was more news from Chicago in the days and weeks that followed, each bringing its own concern. According to the account that has come down in the family, while Alfred was recovering from influenza, he received orders from the military to deploy overseas, still in a weakened condition. Two of his brothers, Michael Jr. and Peter, were already in uniform.

The crushing blow came as fighting escalated that summer. Freddie was grievously injured almost immediately upon entering the zone of combat. He would spend most of the next year in a French hospital, too weak to return stateside.

For Pierre and Mary, bitter irony added to their concern for Freddie. The Sartor and Winandy families had left Europe for a better life in America. Now Mary's brother was lying in a hospital not far from their homeland.

Pierre was under a great deal of strain. He was middle-aged and at the midpoint of his career, a time in life when many men and women feel intensified pressure. Pierre was responsible for a large family and was the sole physician for hundreds of towns-folk and farmers across a wide rural area. And he was starting a new practice amid the emerging threat of a pandemic.

In the spring and summer of 1918, Pierre and other doctors read about the novel strain of influenza that was making its way through military camps and cities. Questions arose in the medical community: *How did it spread? What direction would it take? Could it be stopped?*

Compounding the complexity for doctors, who probed the disease while the nation focused its resources and will on the war effort, was the fact that, at this stage, not everyone agreed the influenza outbreak was a crisis. While young adults were indeed dying of the condition, even greater numbers became ill and recovered. Depending upon one's perspective at this juncture, the new type of influenza might be the equivalent of a rampaging plague, or just a nasty "three-day fever." The Sartor family's experience mirrored this ambivalent picture. Freddie had taken ill, and influenza was circulating in the Midwest — but Mary and Guido still made their trip to Chicago.

It is impossible to know Pierre's thoughts about the influenza outbreak at this time. In one sense, he may have been ahead of some of his peers. Having grown up in Luxembourg, Pierre had a deeply rooted perspective that encompassed much of Western Europe, augmented by his medical studies and personal empathy for people, especially the poor, who became caught in the onslaught of illness. Informed by historical memory that spanned generations, Pierre knew that outbreaks of disease often came in waves.

This, in fact, was the course that the influenza pandemic followed.

To understand Pierre's actions in the months that followed, it helps to give his story context. The Centers for Disease Control and Prevention identifies three phases of the influenza pandemic, with the caveat that the timing and impact of the successive waves varied among geographic locations.

The first phase occurred from March through the late summer of 1918. Early outbreaks in Kansas spread unevenly across the United States to Europe — facilitated by large-scale troop deployment — where it acquired the nickname "Spanish flu" and reached other places around the world. While the disease remained prevalent in many locations, there was a general sense that the influenza was subsiding by the late summer.

The second phase began with an explosive outbreak in Boston in September 1918. A more virulent strain of the disease, this form of influenza spread rapidly and claimed the greatest number of deaths before subsiding toward the end of the year.

The third phase of the influenza pandemic, according to the CDC, began in early 1919. It, too, was highly lethal; flu-related deaths continued, albeit in diminishing numbers, into the summer.

Precise statistics are unavailable, but the pandemic caused about 50 million deaths around the world, including approximately 675,000 in the United States — more than 10 times the number of American combat-related deaths in World War I. Influenza claimed about 6,000 lives in Iowa.

It is remarkable, then, that three phases of the influenza pandemic may also be discerned in Pierre's story. In his case, they were sharply delineated not only by dates but also by specific events including, as we will see, the dramatic arrival of "Patient Zero" into Pierre's community and a "superspreader" event that magnified the number of cases, straining Pierre to the utmost and having significant consequences for his family.

He could not have planned it this way, but his timing was impeccable. For Pierre, the first phase of the pandemic, discussed in this chapter, lasted from early spring 1918 to the end of summer. Through Freddie's illness and what he read and heard during this time, Pierre developed a keen appreciation of the severity of the condition, which had not yet reached the people he served. This was also the period when Pierre moved his family and medical practice to Titonka, the place where he would spend the rest of his life. He had time — barely — to get established before the onslaught came.

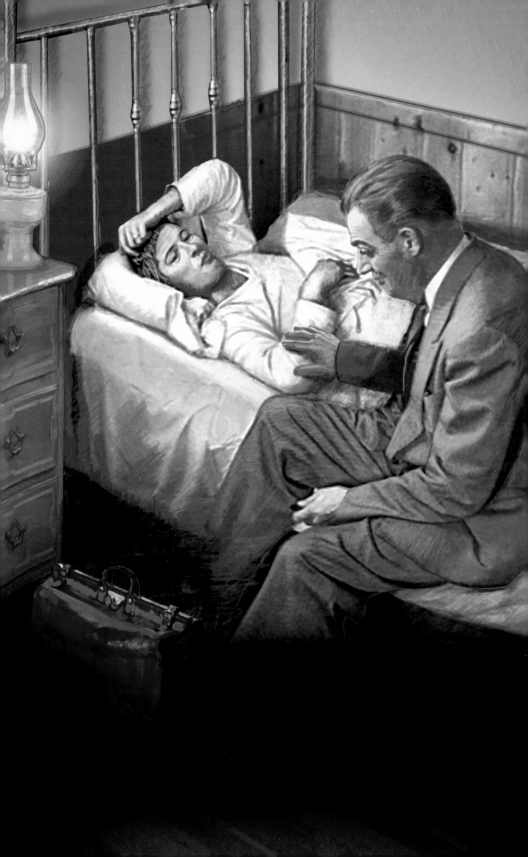

CHAPTER 15

"My 'Flu Life'"

Titonka, Iowa
September 1918

"SUMMER OVER. FALL SEASON HERE, winter just around the corner. And still no 'Flu' as yet."

Thus begins Pierre's first-person account of his fight against the influenza pandemic. The experience was so consuming that he entitled his memoir "my 'Flu Life,'" preceded by words that speak to his excitement at the challenge and his immense dedication to his patients.

The full title of Pierre's narrative is "Thrills of my life — specifically my 'Flu Life.'" He wrote it by hand in 1953; the quotations that follow come from his manuscript and a typed transcription.

Pierre's word choice is interesting, even considering that English was not his first language. (Actually, it was his fifth language, after German, French, the dialect of Luxembourg and Latin.) What did Pierre mean by "thrills"? The fact that he discussed the influenza pandemic, conversationally and in formal

Pierre devoted medical skill, compassion and prayer to his patients during the influenza pandemic and throughout his career.

presentations, for decades afterward shows that the events of 1918-1919 played a central role in his life and self-concept.

I believe that for my grandfather, the "thrill" was his sense of making a difference, of being in the right place — in his oft-repeated phrase, "I am needed" — at the right time.

The fall of 1918 marked a turning point for Pierre as well as for the nation and the world. In its second phase, the influenza pandemic spread rapidly.

The outbreak was devastating where it occurred, but for much of September, Pierre watched the unfolding crisis from afar. From what he read in the news and discussed with his colleagues, including Dr. Wallace, who described his medical experience in service with the military, Pierre understood this was not a typical bout of seasonal flu, nor was it a repeat of the influenza that had reached around the world earlier that year. This outbreak was more widespread — and far more deadly.

Pierre's approach to medicine went beyond treating the patients at hand. He took a broad view and was interested in the cause and diffusion of disease as well as its signs and symptoms. In this regard, one may compare Pierre to Hercule Poirot, the fictional detective created by novelist Agatha Christie around this time. Poirot was from Belgium, near Pierre's homeland of Luxembourg. Both were roughly contemporaries, being in middle age during the World War I era. The resemblances between Poirot and Pierre are striking. Consider this description of Poirot by his fictional companion Captain Arthur Hastings: "He was hardly more than five feet four inches but carried himself with great dignity. . . . His moustache was very stiff and military. . . . The neatness of his attire was almost incredible."

Poirot wore a pocket watch and was meticulously punctual, which is consistent with Poirot's sense of professionalism. Most of all, Poirot solved his cases through deduction and analysis — in his (or, rather, Agatha Christie's) words, making effective use of "the little grey cells" as well as "order and method." This is also an excellent description of Pierre's systematic approach to providing medical care.

Pierre's experience with rural as well as urban living, along with his empathy for the poor and awareness of their suffering from contagious illness, shaped his perspective. He had already concluded that horses, especially their waste and carcasses, were a source of disease. He now theorized that influenza could spread in the air as well as by direct contact with body fluids. Today, we know his conclusion was correct.

Mulling over these thoughts, during the fall of 1918 Pierre began to develop a multifaceted plan to meet the intensifying health crisis. His response was built upon key principles, but he also had the flexibility to adapt his plan to changing conditions. The three pillars of his plan were education, involvement and isolation.

Pierre was determined to educate people about the influenza outbreak. His outreach ranged from one-on-one conversations with patients to commentary he submitted to the *Titonka Topic,* the local newspaper that was established in 1899 and was the primary source of information and social connections for people in town and the surrounding area.

Pierre moved beyond conveying information to engaging the active involvement of his community in fighting the flu. From hygiene to prevent infection to best practices in caring for the ill, Pierre tapped the home-front spirit of World War I to enlist what one could think of as an army of volunteers who would follow his methods and extend his model of care.

In describing the pandemic years later, Pierre repeated the mantra he gave to people at the time: *Stock soap, a lot of soap. And accumulate bedsheets, enough to burn.* These were simple, practical steps that related to daily life, but also called attention to the urgent health condition.

Isolation was central to Pierre's vision for fighting the flu. His belief that influenza spread through the air as well as by direct person-to-person contact drove his determination to separate infected patients from others to minimize the spread of disease. In the weeks and months to come, he would advocate for isolation, and would secure the compliance of his patients and their families to a degree and with a level of success that was unmatched in many other communities.

Pierre's experience aligned with Mayo Clinic's. With good planning and the providence that often attended their efforts, the Sisters of St. Francis in Rochester, Minnesota, opened an Isolation Unit at Saint Marys Hospital in June. This specialized facility was staffed and ready as the pandemic gathered momentum. Indeed, its first patient was associated with the site where the outbreak began. According to the *Annals of Saint Marys Hospital*: "June 14th, the first patient was received, a young soldier from Fort Riley, Kansas."

Titonka, Iowa, had no such advanced medical facility, but its rural lifestyle and widely dispersed population made what later generations called social distancing more feasible.

Pierre began his campaign for flu awareness by targeting the slough. The marshy remains of a preglacial riverbed, it connects two watersheds, the Blue Earth River and the east fork of the Des Moines River. As such, it is a natural habitat for waterfowl, upland wildlife and prairie tallgrass. In 1938, by Executive Order, the area was designated as the Union Slough National Wildlife Refuge; today, it encompasses 3,334 acres of marsh and upland habitat. The U.S. Fish and Wildlife Service offers activities that include hunting, fishing, wildlife viewing, interpretative programs, environmental education and photography.

When Pierre's family moved to Titonka, the slough covered about 8,000 largely unmanaged acres. Attempts over the years to construct levees and ditches had proven futile; because the area was considered unfit for agriculture, it was a popular location for hunting and fishing, and children loved to roam and explore there.

Might the flu spread in water? The *Titonka Topic* readily covered that question. At home, Pierre told his children they could continue their pastime of sloughing — his word for wading through the backwater — just not that autumn. There would be other times in the future.

But this was the Sartor children's first year in Titonka, and oh, the pull of that slough. Going there was just about their favorite recreation. But then, one day it happened: The slough issue was sealed. While out hunting in the backwater, Billy Johnson accidentally put a load of buckshot into a fellow hunter's lower leg. Pierre dressed the man's wound for immediate relief, then sent him to the Algona hospital for follow-up care including removal of wadding, shot and bits of his rubber boots that penetrated his leg where the buckshot tore into it.

The hunting accident inadvertently underscored Pierre's credibility as an advocate for public health and safety. By community consensus, and ultimately by regulation, the slough would be off limits to children each hunting season in the years ahead. For the fall of 1918, this had the immediate benefit of Pierre getting the public's attention and children getting out of harm's way — from buckshot and the contagious spread of influenza.

Pierre tapped several cultural resources in making his case for flu awareness. According to the norms of small-town America at the time, the local doctor was a respected authority figure, often one of the best-educated people in town. The doctor was known to virtually everyone, by first-person experience as patients or by word of mouth. Scientific medicine had reached the point where people trusted a doctor's judgment and willingly sought a physician's care. Trust in medicine coexisted with religious faith in many people of the time, creating a foundation for coping with crises like the influenza pandemic. This, too, was an advance from Pierre's youth, when illness was often interpreted as punishment for sin.

Pierre's individual situation also equipped him as a leader. A man of deep faith and useful skills, with empathy for the poor and suffering, he felt a strong conviction to serve his people. He was new in town, offering a fresh perspective amid rapidly changing conditions without the baggage of past experiences and entrenched relationships that might limit a doctor of long tenure in the community. Pierre avoided conflict, using charisma and charm to help make his case to reluctant patients. He had the confidence of a seasoned professional in the prime of his career; his approach to caring for patients was enriched by insights from his network of other Iowa physicians and his connections to regional hospitals and Mayo Clinic. And, as the only physician in Titonka and the surrounding area, he had autonomy and freedom to act.

Yet even Pierre could only do so much. With no flu in town, life went on. The *Titonka Topic* shows, for those weeks in the early autumn, people were more interested in local issues and the far-off war than in the form of influenza that was churning through the country.

That autumn, Guido readied the car for the cold weather to come. An older high school friend, Bub Ribsamen, "keen on cars and radios," as Guido would later describe, helped him work on the vehicle. Guido described how they "rigged" the car, spacing its wheels farther apart, so it could travel along in the ruts of snow made by bobsleds. They nicknamed the car "The Riggedy-Jig."

Some days the boys drove to the rural areas around Titonka for a picnic. On Sundays in fair weather, Pierre took Mary or one of the children on a motoring trip through the countryside. If they passed a car, they got smothered in dust, of course, but Mary was accustomed to shaking the skirts of her travel suit and the children looked at such events as an adventure.

As the weather turned cooler, Mary buckled down. She had knitting and sewing quotas to meet for the Red Cross. She received a glowing evaluation for her handiwork. Mary and her friends met their requirements for split irrigation pads (for surgery), operating aprons and caps, pajamas and bed shirts. Sweaters were tied in bundles of five.

Always frugal, Mary scrimped even more, given the shortages that consumers faced in wartime. She followed the Native Americans' way. If patients paid their medical bills with a killed animal, it was not used just for food; Mary saved the fur

The Sisters of St. Francis opened an Isolation Unit at Saint Marys Hospital in June 1918. As recorded in the Hospital Annals, it was ready for the first patients with influenza, who arrived soon after.

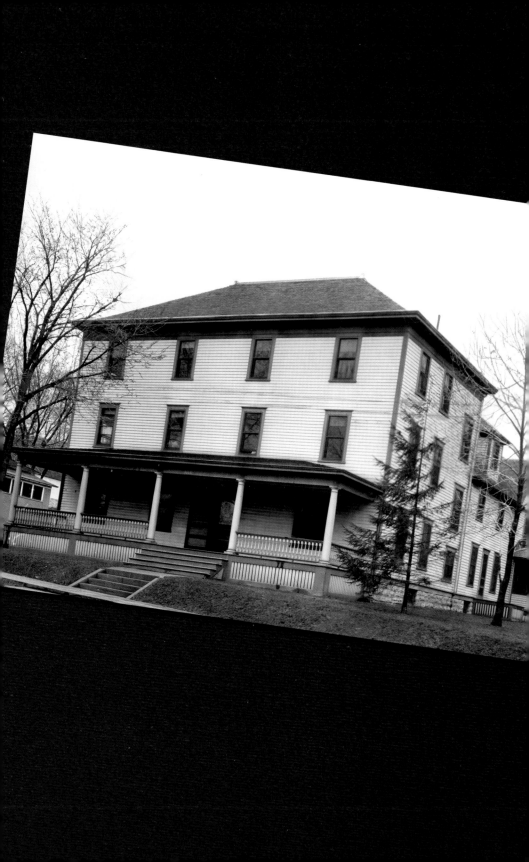

or feathers, as well as the organs, because the entire animal should be used. Mary made lung soup for supper, using a recipe from Luxembourg. In the upper left-hand corner of her recipe card, she hand-painted a flower.

Pierre and Mary's older daughters joined the Canning Club; most girls did. The *Algona Courier* encouraged girls to enter their goods at the Kossuth County Fair, where Canning Club teams competed. The Kossuth County Farm Bureau had been established the previous year and in 1918 enrolled 57 boys and girls in three clubs, including the newly established dairy calf club.

A woman in Algona wrote up directions for canning with wartime wisdom. Because sugar was in short supply, she urged thrifty homemakers to use glycerin from buckthorn bushes. At the time, buckthorn was an imported and desirable ornamental shrub. And so, Girl Scouts in uniform went all over town, identifying this new designer shrub. In time, buckthorn became invasive, creating an environmental menace that in some ways paralleled the consuming spread of influenza throughout the country.

Meanwhile, folks socialized, interacted. Children started school, including all the Sartor children, except Anthony, the youngest. Pierre watched Anthony's health carefully. His breathing was labored.

In the mornings, Pierre went to his office on Main Street to attend his patients. Some accounts have come down to us: A farmer was rushed to Pierre, on a wagon pulled by two mules, his foot propped on a crate. He'd been caught in a windmill. In their haste to extricate the farmer and seek Dr. Sartor's help, his rescuers pulled the man out of his trousers, leaving them to flap in the breeze as the windmill blades went round and round. Pierre tended to cases like this, and many others more mundane, as the flu took hold elsewhere.

Did Pierre feel anxiety or frustration as he followed news of the spreading influenza? It must have been challenging for him to encounter local perceptions that ranged from *It won't happen here* to *We can't do anything about it, anyway* to *It's in God's hands.* Fatalism, resignation, denial and blind faith were not part of his thinking, or consistent with the practical measures he formulated to defend the community.

Pierre also knew that while he was making plans, other doctors were immersed in the crisis. His medical school classmate John Dill Robertson was the Health Commissioner for Chicago. He had held the position since 1915 and now led the influenza response of one of the nation's largest cities. The second wave of influenza struck Chicago on September 8, when several sailors at the nearby Great Lakes Naval Training Station reported being ill. The disease spread quickly among other military units in the area and entered the civilian population, which put the Winandy and Sartor families, and Pierre and Mary's many friends in High Ridge, at risk. Dr. Robertson made influenza a reportable disease on September 16. As influenza surged in the days and weeks that followed, recalled Morris Fishbein, M.D., a prominent Chicago physician and longtime editor of the *Journal of the American Medical Association*, Chicago doctors visited between 60 and 90 patients a day.

There is a plaintive tone in Pierre's memoir when he wrote of this time:

> *'My God,' I was a-thinking, did the Lord forget me?*
> *No case as yet. I could diagnose a 'flu.'*

Pierre did not have long to wait. The fact that Titonka had so far escaped influenza made the ever-closer occurrences seem like the inexorable advance of an invading army, a vivid image for many people after four years of the Great War. Pierre wrote:

> *Travelling salesmen telling stories of flu, funerals every day only some 10-20 miles away. Towns quarantined, no one stayed in this or that town no longer than absolutely necessary.*

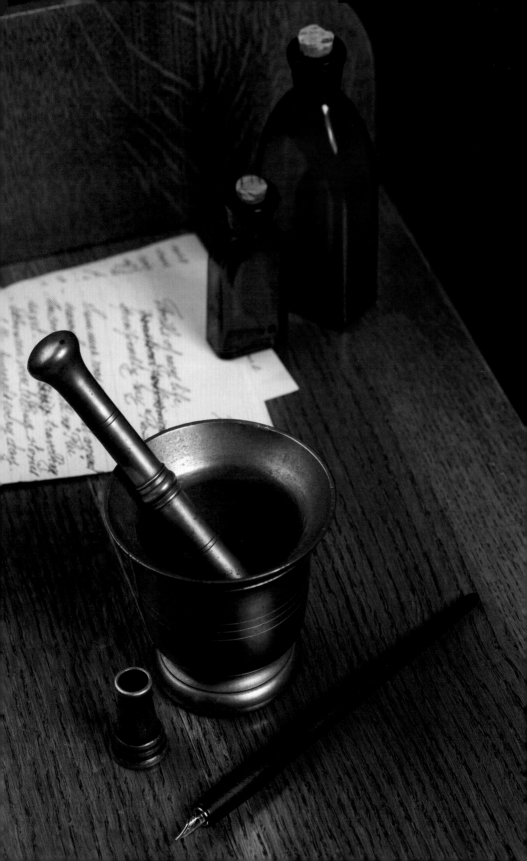

CHAPTER 16

"Here was the long-expected 'real Flu'"

Titonka, Iowa
October 1, 1918

WITH INFLUENZA BREAKING OUT around much of the world, it was difficult — at that time and even today, in retrospect — to chart the rapid progress of the disease. In this context, Pierre's experience was distinctive. For the population he served, he not only knew the first person to have symptoms, but also documented the patient's name and case history.

It was a train that brought influenza to Titonka:

> *Then — on the first of October, Mrs. Geo. Lamoreux came home on the 'Klondike' around 5 o'cl in the afternoon. A mighty sick woman.*

Timing is symbolic. According to the Centers for Disease Control and Prevention, October 1918 was one of the deadliest months in U.S. history, "when approximately 200,000 Americans died of the flu. Healthy young adults (average age 35 years) began coughing in the morning and were dead by evening. The family stories . . . define true courage amid unbearable loss."

Pierre was summoned from his office when the first patient with influenza reached Titonka.

This statement in Pierre's narrative about "my 'Flu Life'" is significant on several levels. Rare among medical accounts of the 1918-1919 influenza pandemic, he pinpointed "Patient Zero" of his practice, a medical term for the first person identified as being infected with a communicable disease. It also happened that, following the pattern of much of his life, Pierre was in the right place at the right time. A savvy career move put him there.

For Titonka and its surrounding area, Dr. Sartor was the official physician of the Chicago, Rock Island and Pacific Railroad Company — known in everyday parlance and a popular folk song, which has been recorded in multiple versions over the years, as the Rock Island Line.

Becoming the designated physician for the Rock Island Line, a position he held for decades, was a career milestone for Pierre. It provided reliable income, since trains at that time were the principal means of long-distance travel.

Guido and Mary's motor trip from Iowa to Chicago across virtually unmarked roads was notable for being a novelty, and commercial passenger air travel of any significance would not start until after the war. Iron rails, far more than highways and airfields, linked the nation together at this time.

Large numbers of passengers and crew members aboard the trains meant that illness of one kind or another would inevitably occur, so railroads contracted with a network of physicians along their routes to provide care as needed. This meant that Pierre saw more patients and a wider range of medical conditions than he would have encountered in a strictly community-based practice.

By seizing the opportunity to work for the Rock Island Line, Pierre displayed initiative akin to that of the Mayo brothers in Rochester, Minnesota, who were appointed as consulting physicians to the Chicago & North Western Railroad early in their careers. According to biographer Helen Clapesattle:

> *The successive developments in transportation have been essential in the Mayo rise, and the first of these was the railroad. When the Mayos were ready for ex-*

pansion beyond the radius of team-and-wagon trav-
el, the rails were ready to provide transportation to
carry the surgeons out and the patients in.

The "Klondike" that Pierre wrote about was a train on the line's regular service. Its name evoked the excitement of the Alaska Gold Rush of the 1890s. In the Pacific Northwest, the Klondike Mines Railway carried treasure; on this date in Iowa, the Rock Island Klondike brought disease.

From Pierre's written narrative in "my 'Flu Life'" and the memories he often shared with family, friends and journalists, it is possible to envision his most memorable experience as the local doctor for the Rock Island Line.

Pierre's office door slammed open. His visitor came direct from the train, through a downpour, and couldn't sit. He talked fast. A lady on the train had taken sick and the presence of illness — this "bug" — looked serious enough to report. Could Doc come along, take a look?

Pierre asked questions; the answers were grim. Pierre listened with an increasing sense of foreboding. He would remember the image of that man, of coal dust dripping from his clothing to the floor — ominous, just by its darkness. As the grime settled, it outlined his footprints on Mary's rag rug.

Pierre realized that an ill passenger could spread disease in the community. It was time to put his plan into action. The first step was to see the patient aboard the train.

Fastidious as always, Pierre pumped water at the office sink and scrubbed his own rough hands, parched dry from the crisp air and the strong soap he used. Pierre grabbed his doctor bag and plucked his coat from a wooden tree in the corner, which Guido had built in shop class.

Pierre was alert and ready. He may have thought, as he often said when expressing his simple but deep faith: *If the Good Lord so will.*

Pierre's office door had a lock. He fastened it because he had no sense of when he would return. A bell rope hung outside his door, placed there for him to pull when he wanted a buggy, horse and driver from the livery stable. He pulled the rope and waited a moment, but then he knew — he couldn't wait. Pierre called to a youngster down the street. He was heading to the train station; when the buggy arrived at his office, the child should have the driver catch up.

That day, he would recall, he wasn't quite dressed for the weather and his visitor was even less protected, wearing bib overalls that flapped in the chilly rain. They hiked double-quick to reach the Klondike. When they got aboard, Pierre made his way through the passenger section, swiping water from his coat.

Mrs. George Lamoreux, as Pierre called her, according to the norms of the time when a married lady was known by her husband's first as well as his last name, is the only patient identified by name in Pierre's memoir. According to genealogical records, it is likely that her full name was Myrtle Harriet Plum Lamoreux (1892-1983), who married George Lewis Lamoreux (1886-1960) in 1911.

Along with describing her as "a mighty sick woman," he documented how she became ill: "She had been visiting her brother in the navy at the Great Lakes navy station, a short distance north of Chicago on Michigan Lake shores."

The first outbreak of influenza in the Chicago area that fall occurred at Naval Station Great Lakes, the U.S. Navy's largest training installation. The facility had opened in 1911 with accommodations for 1,500 sailors-in-training. By the fall of 1918, with America's wartime mobilization at its peak, its population swelled to more than 45,000. Overcrowded conditions proved an ideal venue to circulate that year's form of influenza, which struck otherwise healthy young adults with brutal force.

Although leave was canceled for enlisted men at Great Lakes, influenza spread beyond the base because visitors were still allowed to come and go. Mrs. Lamoreux's case shows how influenza, aided by a mobile population and an efficient national network of transportation, could move swiftly from a major urban area like Chicago to a remote town like Titonka.

Writing of her brother at Great Lakes, Pierre said, "He had the flu, and the train men were positive she had the flu." In the parlance of railroad crew from that era, it was clear that Mrs. Lamoreux would be "on the shelf" (their term for staying in bed) for a long time.

Pierre's immediate challenge was what to do with his patient. In short order the horse and buggy he had summoned from the livery stable arrived. Where to take her? The nearest hospital was in Algona, about 15 miles away, over rural roads — a significant journey for a healthy person making a social call, to say nothing of the "mighty sick woman" who desperately needed care.

As a country doctor, Pierre was comfortable with the fact that most medical treatment took place at home. But even getting Mrs. Lamoreux to her house was out of the question: "Her condition was such, it was judged, she could not be taken to her house a mile southeast of town."

Fortunately, her mother-in-law lived nearby. Hence the decision "to take her to grandma L. house only 2 blocks southeast of depot."

Then, and in retrospect, Pierre knew his time had come: "I was called and here was the long expected 'real Flu.'" He escorted Mrs. Lamoreux from the train, loaded her aboard the buggy and tucked a blanket about her.

"For 3 weeks almost every day I had to be in attendance," he wrote. Pierre's method of caring for Mrs. Lamoreux serves as a case study for his approach with other influenza patients. Through Pierre's recollections and oft-told family stories, one can discern his methodology. He seamlessly blended the art as well as the science of health care.

By bringing Mrs. Lamoreux to her mother-in-law's home, Pierre applied his philosophy of isolating the patient and focusing duties on one caregiver, all with the goal of minimizing the spread of a highly communicable disease. The patient's husband, George Lamoreux, took up residence in an upstairs bedroom. Their children stayed with neighbors who were healthy.

Pierre had a sign painted for the front door, white letters on black: FLU WITHIN/DO NOT ENTER. He achieved a high level of compliance from the community. On the times he came to the Lamoreux house, he noted the calling cards that friends had left on a bench in the hall near the front door. Each represented a small victory in his campaign for isolation since the individual whose name was printed on the card had dropped off this token in lieu of a personal visit.

Family, friends and neighbors also wrote notes and sent flowers. They brought books with dried flowers poking from between the pages. Toys appeared by the doorway, all boiled or washed, a loan to the Lamoreux children. Many people of the time had small leather-bound keepsake albums, and Mrs. Lamoreux's friends wrote messages and get-well sentiments in hers, providing a welcome distraction for the patient.

George's mother, known in Pierre's record as "Grandma L." and "the grandmother," became the principal caregiver. Genealogical records indicate that her full name was Jennie Isenberger Lamoreux (1854-1931). Grandma Lamoreux read notes and letters aloud to her daughter-in-law, keeping her spirits up, and prepared food. Cooking for the ill required extra effort. Pierre's maxim: A patient starts with a carbonated bubbling drink, but not until two full hours after vomiting, and the drink was to be at room temperature, neither hot nor cold. And not another thing by mouth until that first beverage stayed down for four hours. Only then could the patient move on to broth. Grandma Lamoreux could make her finest broth, but she had to cut back on the chicken fat so it would not be over-rich for a convalescing patient.

We do not know if George Lamoreux maintained the discipline of separation from his wife, but toward the end of October, according to Pierre's account, he also "was down" with influenza. In essence, this experience confirmed the wisdom of Pierre's belief in isolation — and the difficulty of achieving it.

In family conversations over the years, Pierre used the understated phrase *a complication* to describe events like the spread of influenza within the Lamoreux household despite his best efforts to contain it. Pierre typically sorted things that happened into categories — *an occasion* or *an incident* for mundane mishaps and irritations, upgraded to *a surprise* or, escalating further, *a bothersome incident*. On rare occasions he might say something was *really an incident*. When Pierre referred to George Lamoreux catching influenza from his wife as *a complication*, the people who knew Pierre realized he viewed it as serious, indeed.

Pierre's care of Mrs. Lamoreux, followed by his care for her husband, represents his first documented mobilization in the fight against the influenza pandemic of 1918-1919. He brought to their case many of the qualities that made him a beloved physician throughout his career.

Pierre came often to the Lamoreux house. He opened the windows to circulate the air in the stuffy bedrooms, even as he wrapped his patients to keep them warm. In his quest for fresh air, Pierre was aided by the unusually warm weather. Except for one freezing blast that came months later, the winter that year was generally mild, and coal-heated homes could maintain their comfort even with the windows open. When Pierre wrote about his "rules" for treating influenza patients, he stipulated: "Windows open. Use of liner shutters, day and night."

As part of his regimen of providing care to Mr. and Mrs. Lamoreux, Pierre modeled the meticulous cleaning that he prized in everyday life and which he strongly urged in the homes of all his patients. He wiped his shoes and eyeglasses, and he insisted on the same treatment for every surface his patients touched.

To Pierre, Mr. and Mrs. Lamoreux were far more than carriers of disease. They were persons of value, with a family. And so, if his first prescription for the flu was isolation, his second was to surround those in his care with warmth and love.

Throughout his career, Pierre had a natural rapport with many of his patients, and that seems to have flourished with how he served Mr. and Mrs. Lamoreux. On a given visit, he might patiently administer their food, spoonful by careful, time-consuming spoonful.

He enjoyed people and could carry on conversations that went well beyond medical topics. Mrs. Lamoreux had contracted influenza from visiting her brother at Great Lakes Naval Training Station. Pierre might have found common ground and a pleasant, diverting topic in discussing Lt. John Philip Sousa, USNR, the director of music at Great Lakes, whose 300-member Bluejacket Band was making a national tour to support Liberty Bond drives. President Woodrow Wilson described the Bluejackets as America's Band. Pierre believed music was good for the spirit and for health. Bands, orchestras and itinerant musicians had been a fixture of his youth in Luxembourg. In his Tonsil Tuesday surgical schedule in Bancroft, he would have encouraged Victrola music or unaccompanied singing to cheer his patients.

One can envision Pierre reading to his patients and making small talk to keep up their spirits. He liked to quote "The Village Blacksmith" by Henry Wadsworth Longfellow: "Under a spreading chestnut tree, the village smithy stands," which evoked the courtyard trees of his boyhood school. Over the course of many years, his family heard — and repeated — the poems and tales with which he regaled his patients.

Sometimes Mrs. Lamoreux, awake too long, would go quiet. She daydreamed. Her eyes circled, fixing upon the doilies on the nightstand, the pattern of the wallpaper or upon Dr. Sartor at her side. Shortly after dusk, Pierre would take the ruby-glass kerosene light from the nightstand out of the room. Darkness encouraged sleep. He had to step carefully to keep the light level stable as he left his patient's room.

Over the days and nights as Pierre attended this couple, the complexion of Mrs. Lamoreux, downstairs, grew quite pink, signifying her gradual return to health. And her husband, sequestered upstairs, gained strength. According to the *Titonka Topic*:

> Geo. Lamoreux called up Tuesday on a business matter and his voice seemed natural. He has had a siege of the 'flu' and he said over the phone that he was weak as a cat. He didn't say which kind.

From what we know, Pierre met the flu and mastered it in his care of Mr. and Mrs. Lamoreux. The question was whether he could sustain that effort among the hundreds of other patients he served across a wide swath of rural Iowa. Pressure was building during the month of October in 1918.

Although Pierre highlighted Mr. and Mrs. Lamoreux in his memoir and prescribed isolation for their care, even at the start of the pandemic in and around Titonka, theirs was not an isolated case.

Other events provide context for the weeks that Pierre cared for Mr. and Mrs. Lamoreux. Consistent with locations throughout the United States and internationally, Iowa experienced early outbreaks of influenza in densely populated locations. At the University of Iowa in Iowa City, word went out: *The campus is now under strict military police security. Anyone entering or leaving campus has to show a pass.* At Iowa State College (today Iowa State University) in Ames, flu patients filled the gym, laid out between hanging sheets that served as barriers between the beds.

Pierre received a telephone call from his colleague and predecessor in Titonka, Dr. Robert M. Wallace, who was stationed at Fort Dodge, north of Des Moines, which experienced a severe outbreak of influenza. The challenge, as Dr. Wallace described it, was to keep the flu out of Des Moines. This was difficult because laborers from Des Moines were working at the fort to expand its facilities in response to wartime demands. As with the experience of Mrs. Lamoreux at Great Lakes Naval Station near Chicago, visitors to Fort Dodge took the infection back with them when they returned home. Streetcars — the main form of public transportation in Des Moines and many cities — were packed to capacity to accommodate the rush of workers. The close, crowded conditions were an ideal breeding ground for infection.

Influenza — both in actual cases beyond Mr. and Mrs. Lamoreux and in heightened awareness of the risk — reached Titonka in these weeks and roused the community's attention, building upon Pierre's warnings. October 15 and 16 brought a cascade of events to the small town. Quarantine was decreed at homes where the disease occurred. The local schools closed to avert the disaster looming at colleges and universities across the state. Pierre supported these directives. He knew that students in a classroom — his own children among them — drank from the same tin cup. With the emphasis he placed on stopping the spread of germs, it made sense to put public education on hiatus.

On October 17, 1918, the *Titonka Topic* published a serialized article from the U.S. Public Health Service entitled "Uncle Sam's Advice on Flu." It dismissed the widespread notion of Spain being the point of origin for the disease and carried a stern admonition:

> *If the people of this country do not take care, the epidemic will become so widespread throughout the United States that soon we shall hear the disease entitled American influenza.*

In Rochester, Minnesota, Pierre's friends and colleagues were undergoing a similar experience:

> *"And then came the influenza epidemic!" So sooner or later says anyone who talks about the war years at the Clinic. They had only thought they were busy before, for now the people literally poured into the Clinic from the immediate community. Assigned duties and stations were forgotten, and every doctor, nurse, technician, and secretary worked wherever he was needed most at the moment, often until late at night. Relatives or friends with any time to spare were called into service, Dr. Will's younger daughter Phoebe among them. The doctors worked on the Clinic floor until four or four-thirty and then started out on drives through the countryside, sending the worst cases they found to the isolation unit at St. Marys.*
>
> *. . . The disease broke out in a mild form in the town first, then suddenly and virulently in the hospital itself. One day in early October, twenty persons, eighteen of them nurses, had to be moved to the isolation house. The next day patients began arriving from all over the community, and within a week the new unit was packed, even to cots in the hallways.*

For the Franciscan Sisters, the pressure was crushing.

> *The Sisters in charge [of the hospital] were in great straits. ... There was a shortage of nurses contingent on the illness of so many at one time ... [Mother Superior sent a request] to offer special prayers for the speedy recovery of Sister Constance and Sister Clarita who are dangerously ill with Spanish influenza, and also for Sister Wendelin whose condition is serious; and that God may avert the epidemic from all the members of our Congregation and all persons in our institutions, and may spare all our Sisters to us.*

Pierre's caseload ticked steadily upward as October wore on:

> *Soon after the Lord sent me the first case, my daily routine was like this: After breakfast left home and made house after house, farm after farm, until about 10 o'cl at night or midnight, home and dinner past twelve, bedtime sleep and usually telephone call answers in bed for new cases giving general behavior directions and promise for next day.*

"The Lord sent me the first case" — Pierre's description of influenza as divine visitation is telling. To Pierre, the pandemic was a calling. In the Bible, Abraham, Jacob, Moses, Samuel, Isaiah and Ananias all heard a divine summons and answered "Here I am" as an expression of commitment to do their part by following God's will. Pierre had a similar view of medicine as his mission, whose apogee came during the influenza pandemic. Pierre integrated personal faith with well-honed skills in scientific medicine.

His anguished cry early in the memoir, "'My God,' I was a-thinking, did the Lord forget me?" now had its answer.

XII
mother and mother
~ at the house

I

Thrills of my life.
~~practical~~ ~~my~~ ~~visional life~~.
specifically my "Flu Life"

Summer was over. Fall
season here. winter just around
the corner. And still no "Flu"
as yet. ~~that day~~ travelling
salesmen were telling stories
of flu. funerals every day.
only some 10-20 miles away.
towns quarantined, no
one stayed in this or that town
no longer than absolutely necessary. "My God", I was athin-
king, did the Lord forget me.
No case as yet I could imagine
a Flu! Then — on the first
of October. Mrs Geo Lamo-
reux. came home on the

CHAPTER 17

"Somehow it spread like wildfire on wild prairie land."

Titonka, Iowa
November 1918-January 1919

FUTURE GENERATIONS WOULD CALL IT A "SUPER-SPREADER EVENT." An analysis of Dr. Sartor's career would align it with phase three of the influenza pandemic as demarked by the Centers for Disease Control and Prevention, when the illness accelerated beyond his power to contain it.

In Pierre's own words, however, it was simply "a barn dance."

> *Somewhere northeast of town there had been a barn dance, and a goodly visited affair. The next day a young farmer, owner of the place felt sick while working hay for a neighbor, taken home, doctor called. "Flu," no doubt, died 3 days later. A couple of children, same flu, got well.*

And from this event, Pierre reported: "Somehow it spread like wildfire on wild prairie land."

Were Pierre and Mary, and perhaps their children, invited to

Pierre's handwritten memoir describes the rapid spread of influenza and his effective means of fighting it.

attend the barn dance? We cannot be sure. But from his years among the farms and small towns of Iowa, Pierre could readily imagine the event without having been there in person. An autumn evening . . . the gathering of widely scattered country folk, eager to see each other . . . drawn into the barn by fiddle music, lanterns and food . . . not to mention whisky, whether it was served openly or whether bottles and flasks were passed surreptitiously from hand to hand with a knowing look . . . people dancing in groups and couples in close embrace . . . teens and young adults heading off to dimly lit corners . . . and the warm, moist air that circulated among them all.

Whereas his description of providing care to Mr. and Mrs. Lamoreux has personal details of individual patients he identified by name, Pierre's narrative of the barn dance is an example of epidemiology on the prairie. Epidemiology is the "big picture" study of the causes, frequency and patterns of a disease process that affects a defined population.

> The place was northeast. The barn dance participants were all from north-east and south-east. Inquiry of names, and sure, most of them came down. The list was a sure guide before time of next break outs in farm places, not only listed and timed ones beforehand, but other victims in the same farm house, north-east, south-east.

Pierre's memoir has a folksy style, but it presents a solid example of geographic- and event-based contact tracing. One can infer that he acted with speed. It is likely that Pierre learned that the host of the dance became ill "the next day" and realized the potential spread of "'Flu' no doubt" to the other attendees. "Inquiry of names" describes Pierre's documentation of persons at risk; "sure, most of them came down" is his record of cause and effect.

When making this assessment, Pierre was not merely reactive. To anticipate the spread of influenza, he used the list of guests at the dance as "a sure guide before time of next break outs." Pierre went further and charted the course of contagion beyond those who personally attended to "other victims in the same farm house." This line of inquiry became part of Pierre's model of care. He would ask patients: *Where have you been? Who have you been with?*

Pierre's description of the barn dance and its aftereffects, however, is more than a set of cold data points. He included details that add a human touch. The focal point of his commentary is "a young farmer, owner of the place" — the father of "a couple of children," a man who spent one day extending hospitality to guests and the next day "working hay for a neighbor." After more than a century, it is worth pondering the grief this young man's family and friends felt when illness suddenly struck a vibrant, well-liked member of the community, and the enduring sense of loss when he "died 3 days later."

In fairness, there was nothing intrinsically wrong about holding the barn dance; absent the pandemic, it would probably have been harmless from a public health perspective. Barn dances were woven into the communal fabric of people's lives. As announced in the *Titonka Topic*: "There is to be a barn dance Thursday night, Oct. 3, in the Ed Huber barn. Everybody invited." The invitation had a patriotic as well as a social incentive, since money donated that night was used to purchase Thrift Stamps for the war effort.

If not a dance, other events that autumn were just as likely to spread influenza — a sewing circle, for example, or the routine get-together to sex chickens (that is, the identification of newborn chicks by gender).

At this point in Pierre's narrative, the focus shifts. He has taken the reader from a crisis on the horizon — "travelling salesmen telling stories of flu" — to when "the Lord sent me the first case," Mrs. Lamoreux, and then to "a goodly visited affair," the barn dance that spread influenza "like wildfire on wild prairie land." Now he described how his beloved hometown — *My Titonka* as he often called it — was consumed by the pandemic:

> *In the meantime the Flu spread in town. Almost every residence, and there were about 60 residences. From town the epidemic was carried to the south and*

south-west, to Doan and further from the town to the north and north-west. When it tapered off in one direction, it would be worse in some other direction. In November the north-east and east there were about 50 farm residences which I would have on my daily list and route.

Another factor compounded the challenge Pierre was facing. The weather in his part of Iowa was unusually mild and wet that winter. According to climate modeling studies, two types of conditions are ideal for promoting transmission of influenza virus: cold-dry and humid-rainy. This linkage would not be confirmed until decades later, but it underscores the results he achieved in saving lives. Pierre faced a perfect storm of a new, virulent strain of influenza and ideal climate conditions for it to spread.

Practicing in a sparsely populated area, Pierre knew he could not combat influenza — much less deal with the other illnesses and accidents that were part of daily life, pandemic or not — by himself. During this time of crisis, Pierre began to apply principles of *scalability*. As an industrial term, this refers to handling a growing amount of work by adding resources to a system, thereby achieving increased yield.

The Mayo brothers used this model to build their medical enterprise. Furthering their ideals of serving patients and advancing medical science, Dr. Will and Dr. Charlie Mayo employed industrial principles to expand their staff and extend their reach. Pierre took a remarkably similar approach: As a solo practitioner, he established a network of volunteers to care for patients according to his methods of isolation and cleanliness. He encouraged volunteers by sharing his belief that when good people get together to make a difference, good things happen.

Pierre recruited two types of volunteers — those who would provide care for patients in an infected household and those who would provide shelter for the healthy members of a patient's family to limit the spread of disease.

In this effort, Pierre was both challenged and supported by

the norms of small-town and rural Midwestern life in the early 20th century. Sociability was key to their culture. For decades, the *Titonka Topic* reported on the most prosaic comings and goings: who took an auto trip, who visited whom for Sunday dinner. Family and friends "dropped by" each other's houses and received a warm welcome in the front porch, parlor or kitchen; well-wishers crowded a sickroom, providing comfort if not always effective help. They expressed love through personal attendance. People supported one another because it was inevitable that they, in turn, would need support. It was how folks coped with challenges.

Case by case, one by one, Pierre dealt with these natural instincts of his patients and their loved ones. As he wrote:

> *Right here let me mention one of my rules strictly enforced if possible was 'isolation,' no 2 patients in any one room and much less in one bed.*

Despite the limited state of medical knowledge at the time, Pierre's advocacy for isolation was an effective measure to disrupt the spread of influenza. The disease can be transmitted in a variety of ways: as invisible airborne particles expelled during breathing by an infected person and inhaled by others; as droplets sprayed via talking, sneezing, coughing or other expulsions from an infected person that transfer droplets to another person's mouth, eyes or nose; through hand-to-hand contact from infected people to others who then rub their mouth, nose or eyes; when uninfected people touch contaminated surfaces and then rub their mouth, nose or eyes.

At Mayo Clinic, the Sisters of St. Francis paralleled Pierre's approach to isolation: "As the virulence of the strange disease became better known and mortality from it was increasing, physicians began to require stricken persons to be isolated."

Pierre had to look deep within himself to issue such medical edicts, which impinged upon the daily lives of his patients, because throughout his life he avoided confrontation. But he was a shrewd judge of character and situations and realized that challenges also present opportunities.

Pierre began by identifying individuals to be caretakers. He trained them to go into the home to care for the patient, observing strict hygiene — *Do not touch the patient or anything near the patient more than necessary . . . wash after any contact with the patient.* He took time to get to know each volunteer, assessing the person's strengths and weaknesses. He had to understand, quickly, and play to each person's special abilities.

To make his point about isolation, Pierre spoke in everyday language that people could understand. He used trees as an example. When trees are too close together, their roots become intertwined, causing the trees to die. When trees need sun, the branches naturally lean away from one another.

Isolating the ill was difficult, but Pierre's success in caring for Mr. and Mrs. Lamoreux proved it could be done. A notice in the *Titonka Topic* showed that people were able to accept and apply Pierre's principles, even if it meant temporary separation of family members. A woman identified only as "Grandma Ringsdorf" (first name not needed since most readers in this small town knew her) reported she "spent the last of the week at the home of her son Ross, caring for the baby, absence of Ross and wife [with the flu]."

As to the other group of volunteers, those who would host healthy members of an infected family, Pierre found a ready response. It was natural for people in this culture to "take in" members of the community who could not fend for themselves. The Lamoreux children, for example, lived apart from their parents while Grandma Lamoreux and Pierre brought their mother and father back to health.

Pierre also tapped into the patriotic tenor of the times. World War I was the first large-scale mobilization of the American public in wartime, heavily promoted through patriotic posters, speeches and events. Although separated by an ocean and thousands of miles from the actual fighting, Americans were told they were serving on the home front with the incessant call to take action. This meant purchasing Liberty Bonds; setting aside meat, sugar and other food staples on certain days of the week; and, like Mary Sartor, knitting all manner of goods for the troops and civilians to use. From theaters on Broadway to parlors in Titonka, popular music appealed to wartime sacrifice, urging people to "Keep the Home Fires Burning" in order to help all those who were serving "Over There."

Pierre's call for people in and around Titonka to have sheets enough to burn may have been more evocative than literal, but it fit the context of the times, when the public was focused on "preparedness." Mayo Clinic shared this spirit. Both Mayo brothers served with the U.S. Surgeon General to accelerate medical education for physicians amid wartime demands; Mayo Clinic also collaborated with the University of Minnesota to equip a base hospital and mobile surgical unit on the Western Front in France. In Rochester, Minnesota, the Kahler Corporation established a nursing school (later known as Methodist-Kahler School of Nursing) and Saint Marys Hospital focused its nursing school program to meet civilian and military needs.

Establishing a network of volunteers throughout his territory in rural Iowa did not mean that Pierre was any less involved with direct patient care. His memoir is rich with case studies that provide diverse perspectives on his qualities as a physician and his methods in fighting the pandemic.

Pierre's memoir shows his deep humanity — and a touch of humor. After repeatedly making the point about his "rule" of isolation, he included this account, which shows he could adapt to individual circumstances:

> One married couple with already grown up children. Mother was first, soon followed by husband, one day I found both mother and husband in one and same bed. When I reminded them of my rule of "Isolation," mother said, "Doctor, I rather die of the Flu than to be even a single night without my husband for 30 years[;] we never missed a single night without company to each other." "All right," I said, "no rule without exception, may the good Lord be with you."
> What else could I do?

Pierre's memoir is remarkable for the way he blends health care and human relations into a brief narrative:

*In one farm family there were 3 severe cases. One
downstairs, a grandpa about 75 [years] old who had
pneumonia-flu while upstairs 2 daughters had flu. I
was fortunate to get one of Dr. Dolmage's nurses. It
was hard work for the poor nurse, upstairs, downstairs, and running up and down the stairs. One day,
about the 7th day, I told the nurse, "Girlie, you are
going to have the flu." No, she said, I am not. "Why
not," I said. Well, Dr. Dolmage has vaccinated me
both against the flu and the pneumonia. (There was a
kind of vaccination in those days, I believe the Rosenthal vaccination.) "Good," I said, "but remember
what I tell you now. You will be in bed tomorrow, a
mighty sick girl, when I come back tomorrow." And
so it was. "Now I tell you," I said. "You do not know
me very well. Would you rather have Dr. Dolmage or
myself take care of you." "Well, Doctor Sartor, I do
not have you feel offended, but I rather have Dr. Dolmage take care of me." "Good," I say. "I call him at
once." So I did, the doctor said he could not come at
once, to [too] busy, cannot leave hospital will be there
after one o'cl. All right. I kept on agoing on my daily
rounds and I happened to be at the farm home of my
first Flu patient. The children were having the flu.
Phone rang. Mrs. Lamoreux answered and it was Dr
D at the nurses place. He said, "come at once there is
a mighty sick girl here, your nurse." I did. The nurse
passed away about 9 o'cl that very night. A couple of
days after the old gent passed out a victim of flu
pneumonia, my second loss in the fight.*

This vignette shows Pierre's plan at work. A family, hit hard
by the flu, was practicing isolation — Grandpa in a downstairs
bedroom and two grown daughters upstairs. Other family
members are not described, so one can infer that they, too,
were adhering to Pierre's plan and had relocated to live with
relatives or friends.

Pierre had arranged for a trained caretaker to assist the patients: a nurse who worked for his colleague, Dr. George F. Dolmage, showing the collaborative medical network that supported the rural population. Professional nurses were rare in this area, so it is a sign of the severity of the family's illness that, as Pierre says, "I was fortunate" to secure her services.

Pierre's account also describes the strain upon health care workers as they went back and forth to serve patients. Pierre visited the family but then had to keep "on agoing on my daily rounds." He called Dr. Dolmage for assistance only to hear his colleague say, "to [too] busy, cannot leave hospital." But Dr. Dolmage did not reject Pierre out of hand. Despite the pressure he was under, Dr. Dolmage committed to "be there after one o'cl." Dr. Dolmage reached the farmhouse as promised and then had to call Pierre to return: "Come at once." Without hesitation, Pierre agreed: "I did." The account takes us well into the night of a long day, which would have been one of many.

Of course, the greatest burden fell upon the nurse: "It was hard work . . . upstairs, downstairs, and running up and down the stairs," which went on, one can assume practically without respite, for seven days. Pierre does not tell us how he came to this determination, but with judgment from years of medical practice, he observed the stress the nurse was facing and predicted, "'You will be in bed tomorrow . . . mighty sick.' . . . And so it was."

The give-and-take between Pierre and the nurse is revealing for interactions among health care workers who must care for each other in the midst of medical crises. When Pierre warned her about getting the flu, she stood her ground: "No, I am not." When he asked why, she replied: "Well, Dr. Dolmage has vaccinated me both against flu and the pneumonia." Pierre then added the following commentary: "(There was a kind of vaccination in those days, I believe the Rosenthal vaccination.)"

It is likely that when Pierre referred to "the Rosenthal vaccination," he meant Rosenow's serum, which provides another connection to Mayo Clinic.

The confusion of names — Rosenthal vs. Rosenow — is understandable since Pierre was recounting his conversation with the nurse decades after it occurred. At the same time, this part of his memoir shows Pierre's acuity of mind as he approached his 82nd birthday. It appears he was aware that his reference to the developer of the serum might not be exactly right. In making it, Pierre set his commentary within parentheses to separate it from the main text. He also added an important qualifier: "*I believe* the Rosenthal vaccination" — emphasis added. Pierre's tentative reference stands in contrast to his strong, declarative statements elsewhere in the memoir: "Right here let me say . . . one of my rules strictly enforced. . . "

The serum was named for its developer, Edward C. Rosenow, M.D., head of the Mayo Clinic Division of Experimental Bacteriology.

Born in Alma, Wisconsin, in 1875, Dr. Rosenow was four years younger than Pierre and, like Pierre, received his M.D. in Chicago; in Dr. Rosenow's case, from Rush Medical College. Dr. Rosenow stayed in Chicago after graduation, became internationally recognized in the field of vaccine development and was recruited to Mayo Clinic in 1915. In April 1918, shortly after the first reports of the influenza outbreak, he went to Fort Riley "to make a bacteriologic study of the . . . epidemic."

Dr. Rosenow developed a vaccination (known as "serum" for the fluid component of blood that contains antibodies) that was widely used during the pandemic. Its effectiveness was constrained due to the state of medical knowledge at the time. Viruses — the infective agent in influenza — would not be discovered until the 1930s. Rosenow's serum had some benefit in managing pneumonia, a secondary complication for many patients with influenza in 1918-1919. Pneumonia has a different cause — bacteria — which the medical community was actively studying during the early 20th century.

On December 13, 1918, the *New York Times* reported:

Edward C. Rosenow, M.D., of Mayo Clinic studied some of the earliest cases of influenza and developed a vaccine that was based upon medical knowledge of the time.

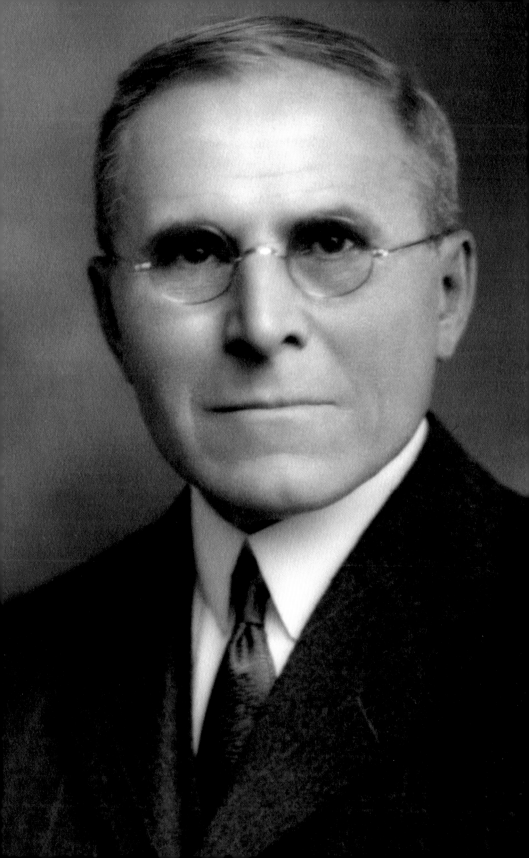

> *Dr. Copeland [New York City Health Commissioner]*
> *. . . was favorably impressed with the vaccine of Dr.*
> *E. C. Rosenow of the Mayo Clinic . . . preparing Dr.*
> *Rosenow's vaccine so it may be given to people of the*
> *city. Rosenow's vaccine was used in Chicago and in*
> *the Middle West on a large scale.*

Anne Brataas, a Minnesota-based medical writer and historian of medicine, science and technology, who has studied and presented on the work of Dr. Rosenow, concludes:

> *Dr. Rosenow had an evidence-based, but unproven*
> *"scientific premonition" of the nature and existence*
> *of viruses decades before their microscopic character-*
> *ization. . . . Rosenow's original view of changeable*
> *bacteria took on new urgency given the public health*
> *emergency of the pandemic — bacteria were acting,*
> *so doctors must too.*

As Helen Clapesattle described:

> *The day after the* Journal of the American Medical
> Association *published Dr. Rosenow's offer to fur-*
> *nish it at the nominal cost of manufacture or to tell*
> *any qualified bacteriologist how to make it, the Clinic*
> *received four hundred telegrams asking for a supply.*

The serum was administered in one, two and three doses. While it may have helped some individuals, as Clapesattle concludes, "the true effect of the shots could not be gauged."

According to an article published by the Iowa State Historical Society:

> *Several vaccines, including one developed at the*
> *Mayo Clinic and tested in Sioux City and Cedar*
> *Rapids, produced uncertain results, but people in the*
> *latter city proved so eager to try it that the demand*
> *for the Mayo vaccine quickly outran the supply.*

The serum did not protect Dr. Dolmage's nurse, despite her confidence in getting the vaccination. She became ill as Pierre had predicted, but a sense of her grit and strength of character comes through Pierre's memoir as she continued the bantering exchange with her employer:

"Now I tell you," I said. "You do not know me very
well. Would you rather have Dr. Dolmage or myself
take care of you." "Well, Doctor Sartor, I do not have
you feel offended, but I rather have Dr. Dolmage take
care of me."

One may discern a sense of relief in Pierre's reply: "'Good,'
I say. 'I call him at once.'"

This story takes another twist — when Dr. Dolmage reached
Pierre, Dr. Sartor was providing care, of all places, "at the farm
home of my first Flu patient." This vignette shows that the tra-
vails of the Lamoreux family had not ended. Pierre wrote, "The
children were having the flu." According to the *Titonka Topic*:

Geo. Lamoreux and family are still down with influ-
enza. They have been having a siege of the trouble.

John Lamoreux spent several days last week in bed
with the 'flu.' He came up town Saturday looking
pretty peaked.

Mrs. Lamoreux, however, was well enough to answer the
telephone and pass along the message from Dr. Dolmage to
Pierre. Pierre arrived in time to attend the nurse at her passing
"about 9 o'cl that very night." The story has further sadness:
"A couple of days after the old gent passed out a victim of flu
pneumonia, my second loss in the fight."

The following account underscores the role of volunteers —
an individual caretaker named Tony and the Red Cross as an
organization — in assisting Pierre:

In another case on the South side of town it took a
special allowance of the Red Cross representative. An
ordinary laborer and his wife came down with the flu
at the same time and of course in the same bed, of
necessity there was only one bed. A man from town
was hired to take care of them. There was also a little
boy about 3 years became sick and of course was in
the same bed nestled between father and wife which
of course exposed the little one from both sides. There
was a children's buggy in the house and I naturally
supposed where there was a buggy there would be a

little pillow and quilt and so on. So I gave the atten-
dant man the order to remove the little boy from be-
tween father and mother to the buggy. I left to go to
the next house. But I was called back by Tony, the
attendant, and he said, "Doctor, there is neither pil-
low, nor little quilt nor anything in the house."
"Tony, I send the Red Cross man down here and you
will get all you need." Good. And all three got along
fine after that.

Along with medical information, the socioeconomic description shows the range of patients that Pierre served. The Lamoreux family had a telephone as well as the time and discretion-
ary means for Mrs. Lamoreux to travel to Chicago; Grandma
Lamoreux lived in a two-story home with enough bedrooms to
accommodate herself as well as her ill son and daughter-in-
law. The "ordinary laborer" and his wife lacked even blankets
for their ill child. We also see the pressures bearing down upon
Pierre. He made the effort to note the living conditions of his
patients, but we can tell he was pressed for time. He spotted
the child's buggy and made a logical assumption: "I naturally
supposed where there was a buggy there would be a little pillow and quilt and so on," and left to see his next patient.

To his patients, during the pandemic and throughout his career, Pierre would often say: *This will pass; have faith.* By com-
bining his natural charisma and medical authority, Pierre was
a steadying presence. But beneath his professional calm, strong
forces were churning.

During the pandemic, it seems that Pierre underwent a kind
of spiritual journey, which enabled him to hold true to his personal beliefs while accepting and encouraging the faith of others. Such a development was remarkable, considering his
background.

Pierre was a devout Catholic at a time when the church he
loved proclaimed itself to be the only true religion. He had
grown up in Luxembourg, where his family and virtually everyone he knew was Catholic. From the parish school in his
village to advanced studies in the capital city, his education

was filtered through Catholic teaching as light passes through a stained-glass window. He settled into the Luxembourg-Catholic enclave of High Ridge, near Chicago, when he came to the United States. Despite the secular nature of his medical training, he affirmed his roots by marrying into the upper reaches of High Ridge society. When Pierre and Mary moved to Iowa, they chose Bancroft with its community of Luxembourg immigrants and a vibrant Catholic church.

Their relocation to Titonka, however, set a new direction. While many people in town spoke German, few hailed from Luxembourg and there was no Catholic church. By accepting the call to practice in Titonka, Pierre opened himself to physician-patient encounters that extended well beyond the parameters he had established in the first decades of his career. The influenza pandemic, coming shortly upon his move to Titonka, greatly accelerated this development, no doubt tapping Pierre's long-held values of tolerance. With illness, anxiety and death around him, Pierre was ever more attuned to the spiritual as well as the medical needs of his diverse patients.

It would have been understandable — and easier — for Pierre to hold his faith as an interior resource and focus on the medical diagnosis and treatment of his patients. Instead, Pierre assessed each situation and when it seemed appropriate, he would ask the patient, if he did not already know: *What might be your religion?* If the patient pursued that line of conversation, Pierre would offer to call in the patient's pastor, whatever the patient's religious affiliation might be; in the meantime, he volunteered to read the patient's choice of prayer.

A Methodist minister, Donald H. James, wrote:

> *Dr. Sartor has had deep respect and confidence from patients of many religious faiths, some of whom were devout Catholics such as he, some who were of other churches but friendly to him and his faith, and some few to whom religion was a barrier but who could still say with the greatest sincerity, "Dr. Sartor is a fine physician and the finest friend a patient could wish." His own fine quality of breadth of culture and*

> *the depth of faith has been summed up by more than*
> *one in Titonka in this way: Because his own faith*
> *means so much, he respects deeply every faith.*

Equally remarkable was the acceptance that Pierre's patients expressed for his faith-based outreach. This was a time when many Protestants harbored deep distrust for the Roman Catholic Church; just a few years later, during the 1920s, the Ku Klux Klan — antagonistic toward Catholics as well as Jews, African Americans and others — would flourish in the rural Midwest. But for Pierre and his patients in the crisis of pandemic, seeds of tolerance were sown.

He also determined to listen to the dying, spending time with them in their final hours. He would administer love even while looking at death. And he would linger alongside the bereaved as well, listening to those left standing around their deceased loved one.

"I will never forget the trust and confidence placed in Dr. Sartor by patients who regarded him as a fine physician and the finest kind of friend," wrote Rev. James.

> *One of these patients . . . having put up a brave*
> *struggle . . . begged of his family and me a special*
> *request, "Tell Dr. Sartor I want to have a long talk*
> *with him about my condition, and I won't ask for*
> *anything more, because I know he won't let me down.*
> *I know he'll do his best for me, because he's my*
> *friend."*

Another person wrote: "He has been a doctor of souls as well as a doctor of bodies with the greatest consideration for everyone and particular favor or prejudice to no one."

As the new doctor in town, he reached out to patients with a modest but well-grounded sense of his own charisma. From his years in Bancroft and his experience since relocating to Titonka, he knew people responded to his energy, skill and dedication. It is likely that he drew upon his own experience of having received help from others. Pierre thought of himself not as a hero, but rather as a bridge who could connect those who need help with what medical science, along with faith and love, could offer.

Pierre began to wear down. He had to try ever harder to disguise his own emotions, which must have been exacerbated by exhaustion. If he couldn't, how could he focus on fighting the flu? How could he be useful to his patients?

It helped Pierre to remember the doctor of his childhood, in Luxembourg. He had gazed into Pierre's eyes, bringing a sense of calm, and the memory stayed with Pierre. That experience had helped shape the way he cared for patients. But this situation was different. As a boy, Pierre had time to heal, with treatment for his ears taking place over nearly a year. In the influenza pandemic, Pierre's patients could die within hours.

Weather conditions added to the sense of misery and uncertainty. The winter was unseasonably mild and, on the many days when it rained, the combination of deluge and pestilence recalled tribulations of biblical proportion.

And then Pierre's workload increased dramatically:

> Doctor Ray in the next town came down with the flu and thus the town and surrounding farm homes came most under my care, a couple of victims in each house, as far as 3 miles east and 4 miles south. Right north of the border of the lake between Woden and Britt . . . where I had 4 flu cases to take care of almost every day.

Pierre's devotion inspired an outpouring of loyalty and respect that extended throughout his career. As one patient wrote: "He was our family doctor when we lived on a mud road far from town, but he never failed to come when called."

This chapter focused on Pierre's care of patients and the scientific methods he used when influenza consumed his region. The next chapter covers the same period with a different perspective — the impact on his community and family. During this time, Pierre encountered an expression among the exhausted people he served, and it is likely he felt the same way himself: *We had the war. We have the flu.*

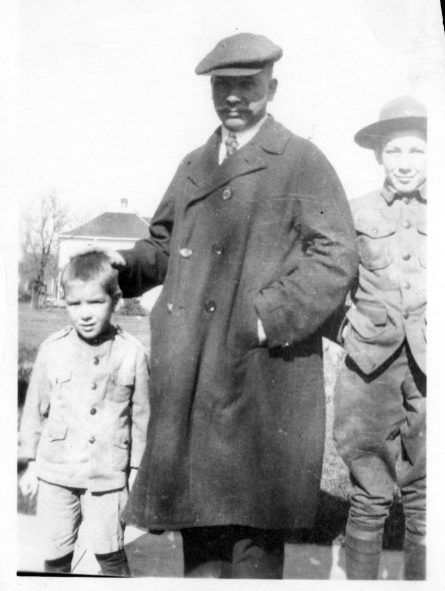

CHAPTER 18

Pierre's Family: Pushed to the Limit

Titonka, Iowa
November 1918-February 1919

"FOR ALMOST THE WHOLE WINTER no fire in the office, nobody to keep it agoing." This reference in Pierre's memoir takes us from seeing him care for patients in their homes to realizing how the pandemic affected Pierre in his own environment — represented by his description of his office, cold and empty more often than not, while he was gone for ever-greater stretches of time.

In a larger sense, Pierre's recollection of a winter with no heat in his office raises the important issue of what happens to health care professionals and their loved ones as they give of themselves to others. Pierre's memoir is the story of one man working against a highly contagious, often fatal disease; it is also important to consider how that dedication took its toll on Pierre and his family.

Many of the following events come from Pierre's written

Pierre and his sons, Anthony (left) and Guido (right), dressed in his Boy Scout uniform, about the time that 12-year-old Guido drove his father to see patients during the influenza pandemic.

memoir as well as the oral traditions of the Sartor family. One especially painful story did not surface until decades later — but after breaking his silence about it, my father, Guido, described the experience so often in his later years that we had to tell him, gently, that we had already heard it.

The relationship between Pierre and Guido took an important new direction at this time, which helped shape Guido's future decision to become a doctor. Pierre made Guido his driver. This action came in response to the fact that more and more, Pierre was arriving home exhausted, having had no rest between his stops at one house or farm after another.

It was a tall order for his 12-year-old son. Guido was at that key juncture between boyhood and young manhood, when impressions and experiences are especially strong. This point of transition is depicted in literary characters as disparate as Jem Finch in *To Kill a Mockingbird*, the Artful Dodger in *Oliver Twist*, Tom Sawyer and Peter Pan.

Guido Sartor's life in rural Iowa was quite different from that of his fictional peers, but he shared with them formative experiences at a crucial time of character development and maturation.

For Guido, it began with helping his father. Pierre needed someone to drive the sleigh, automobile or cart — whatever was the best means of transportation to reach his patients on a given route in whatever the weather might be. Pierre had previously asked friends and neighbors to drive him on an occasional basis. He thought they were saints for helping him out, but this informal approach was episodic and depended upon many variables. Pierre needed a driver he could count on. Guido's mechanical skills and reliability helped confirm Pierre's decision. Who would have guessed that Guido's summertime jaunt with his mother, driving her along dusty roads to Chicago, would set the stage for driving his father through the flu-infested countryside that winter?

Involving Guido was not part of Pierre's original plan. Consistent with Pierre's personality and mission-based view of his profession, his plan was outwardly directed. It focused on his patients: isolating the ill, recruiting volunteers to care for them and providing shelter for their families. The plan included Pierre's increasing commitment to socialize with his patients, engage with their spiritual needs and spend time with the dying even when they were past the point of what medicine could offer. Pierre did all this as a solo practitioner, serving a widely dispersed rural population whose road system and telephone connections were limited even by the standards of the time. He worked during the Midwestern winter of a global pandemic whose end point no one knew. With the expansion of his territory to include Dr. Ray's patients, Pierre was stretched to the breaking point.

In recruiting Guido, Pierre demonstrated the importance of adding inward-directed components to his plan. Just as building a network of volunteers made Pierre's plan *scalable*, ensuring that he had reliable transportation and some chance to rest made his plan *sustainable*.

It seems that Pierre recruited Guido for this role before mid-November 1918. The schools were closed due to the influenza outbreak, so Guido was available. Also, by this time, it must have become clear to Pierre that fighting influenza would be a long-term effort.

The chemistry between them was good. Each knew how the other would react when pushed too far. Swearing or pouting, their needs were transparent.

Now Pierre could visit one patient, go forward, check back. He could respond to change-of-plan appeals from patients, their families and other caregivers, which burst upon his schedule in a variety of ways — perhaps a telephone call or an urgent messenger in a car or sleigh who tracked him down. Pierre could leave Guido to follow through, carrying babies to the next farm and performing other tasks to assist patients and volunteers. Guido's schedule was Pierre's.

Pierre does not mention Guido in his memoir, but the lad, unseen, is there, as Pierre describes visiting "about 50 farm residences which I would have on my daily list and route . . . house after house, farm after farm, until about 10 o'cl at night or midnight." When Pierre left Dr. Dolmage's nurse, only to reverse course and return upon his colleague's summons to "Come at once" and attend her last hours . . . when Pierre departed the laborer's home and was called back by Tony, who was caring for the stricken family . . . in these and other cases, one can imagine young Guido living up to his nickname, Swifty Sartor, adjusting to the sudden changes in plan, getting his father, safely and with dispatch, where he needed to be.

Having Guido as his driver gave Pierre functional, pragmatic help in serving more patients more efficiently. But for Pierre, consciously, and for Guido, probably without his immediate awareness, the new phase in their relationship had additional, deeper meaning. Pierre was a natural teacher, and this highly focused father-son time provided a unique opportunity for mentoring. Pierre's father, Mathias, had set an example of vision and sacrifice for his son, but he could not guide Pierre's professional development, since Pierre attained far more education than Mathias ever achieved. By spending time with Guido, Pierre could fulfill a long-desired transmission of values, knowledge and skills across the generations.

He passed down words of healing to Guido: *This is how you should feel with the flu*, he would say to his patients, addressing his son as well. Meaning: *You are all right.* And this encouraging message for those in his care: *When you get better. . . .*

In this respect, Dr. Sartor was following the pattern of other physicians, including those in the Mayo family. A generation back, Dr. William Worrall Mayo had mentored his young sons, Will and Charlie, on buggy rides to see patients in their homes. According to historian and biographer Judith Hartzell:

> In the traveling classroom, his horse-drawn buggy, W.W. continued educating his sons. At each patient's bedside, he would conduct his routine physical exam under the boys' watchful eyes. Then on the ride home, he helped them draw conclusions from what they had seen.

The traveling-and-mentoring story of Pierre and Guido, however, has more edge. Pierre called Guido to duty at a time of unfolding crisis. Not for them were the relaxing excursions that inspired warm, reflective give-and-take. Father and son were under pressure, coping with wretched conditions as the mud oozed, turning the roads into ruts as hard as bones, and their own health was in danger.

It is worth pondering why Pierre — with his insistence upon isolation — would knowingly, repeatedly expose his son to a lethal disease. Guido did far more than drive. He was often in the sickroom, at Pierre's side, his eyes wide but wise, peeping over a white mask late into night, with contagion ever present.

Under the best conditions, health care workers place themselves in harm's way when serving the ill. This was particularly true as influenza "spread like wildfire on wild prairie land," in Pierre's description. The death of Dr. Dolmage's nurse demonstrates the risk. In one of the stories that follow, we will see how Pierre himself contracted the "dry heaves" from close exposure to a patient.

Mayo Clinic had a similar experience during the influenza pandemic: "The disease broke out . . . suddenly and virulently in the hospital itself. On one day in early October twenty persons, eighteen of them nurses, had to be moved to the isolation house."

The pandemic was no respecter of persons. Dr. Will Mayo wrote to a friend about his brother's illness:

> *Charlie got a cold and bronchitis of the general nature of an influenza-pneumonia, raising a large amount of frothy blood. He arrived from Washington Sunday morning and is just getting around.*

Guido's youth was no protection. Along with healthy young adults and the elderly, children were at great risk in the pandemic. Pierre's memoir describes children who were stricken — youngsters in the Lamoreux family as well as children in other homes. Indeed, perhaps the most poignant experience in Pierre's memoir involves a child he encountered toward the end of the pandemic. The risks to Guido were great.

Although Pierre wrote his memoir in 1953 and the stories have been filtered and retold for generations, it is possible to discern in these events the real-time pressures that he and his family faced.

Outside events bore down upon them. November 11, 1918, brought the Armistice, which concluded hostilities in the Great War. Pierre and Mary could now anticipate the Winandy brothers returning to Chicago.

The youngest brother, Alfred, had been in a French hospital since the past summer. It would have been a great relief to Pierre and Mary to think of Freddie coming home.

Luxembourg, their homeland, which had been under German occupation, was now liberated. General John Pershing, commander in chief of the American Expeditionary Force, issued a statement that "American troops enter the Grand Duchy of Luxembourg as friends, and will abide rigorously by international law." Grand Duchess Marie-Adélaïde, who had protested the German invasion in August 1914 but stayed in the country during the occupation, abdicated the throne in favor of her sister, Charlotte.

The newspapers were filled with reports of celebratory parades, including one in Des Moines, which would have brought back memories of Pierre and Mary's wedding day 20 years before, during the Spanish-American War, when a parade reveled outside their Chicago church. This time was different. Pierre shivered when he thought of the health risk of crowds gathering together.

December — the coming of the holiday season, the end of the year and the shortest days of sunlight — intensified all that was happening around Pierre and his family.

In hindsight, it would be about December 6, St. Nicholas Day by the church calendar and about three weeks after the end of the war, when the mood in Titonka shifted.

Pierre and Guido were going around the clock. Still, everyone wanted to believe that with the fighting over, the flu would surely slow down.

It was not to be. Just when Pierre was seeing cases increase in volume and intensity, the worst turned unimaginable. Between elation over the war's end and the children's celebration of St.

Nicholas Day, his townspeople seemed to lose their sense of caution. They were tired of the flu. Surely, surely, they could go out? And with that, they ventured out and about. They were desperate — for fresh air, for freedom, for a respite to forget the flu. Eager to mix socially, people in Titonka concocted ways to defend themselves against infection. But unlike Pierre's plan of isolation and hygiene, these efforts did nothing to slow the spread of disease.

It was common at the time for people to turn to elixirs and potions that were advertised in newspapers and other publications: "Magic Beans, Brain Powder, Rutabaga: The Path to Eternal Wisdom." Some people used home remedies or improvised their own preventive measures. They applied an onion poultice to their chest or carried a slice of raw potato in their pocket. Pierre arrived at one house to find that a man had tied a string on a rag dipped in turpentine, swallowed it, then pulled it back up his throat. *A close shave*, Pierre said. It was a measly joke, he knew, but if he couldn't use humor as an outlet, he didn't know what to do.

Proof the solve-it-yourself approach became accepted: People who were out and about boldly reported their adventures to the paper. The residents — bragged! The *Titonka Topic* featured a column titled "Happenings of the World, Tersely Told." The December 12, 1918, issue carried these reports:

> *Autoed to Algona on a Santa Claus tour.*
> *Took a load of Burt people to Algona . . . for sight-seeing and shopping.*
> *Went to Woden to visit relatives who are down with the flu.*

At least the school stayed closed, "until December 30 or further notice," according to the *Titonka Topic*. And the bad weather began to help Pierre's cause. The mud was deep. He could only hope that people would stay home. The paper reported that Archie Cunningham "called up from Britt that he is home for the holidays and his father [would have] visited from Titonka but he could not, the condition of the roads." However, some people still got out, including those who attended "a siren of a yard sale on a farm." They walked or rode horseback: "Boys hiked when there were no teams or autos running between towns." The reports had a sense of giddiness: "The corn could be seen, coming up in December. . . . The fields sprouted with weeds. Just the right thing for the farmers, at least."

This mindset terrified Pierre. The midst of the flu was no time to drop one's guard. Pierre followed the comings and goings of his neighbors and patients. Fortunately, he had trained them to wash their hands, which he hoped would help — if they listened.

Then the mail service, the principal form of communication across distances, stopped. "The mail carrier, Mrs. E. J. Hackersbin, is quite ill," said the paper. The unofficial motto of the U.S. Postal Service is "Neither snow nor rain nor heat nor gloom of night stays these couriers from the swift completion of their appointed rounds" — words that had been carved in stone above the door of the New York General Post Office just four years before. Now, what weather conditions could not halt, influenza did. With Mrs. Hackersbin out of commission, there would be no mail between Wesley and Titonka. No mail carrier meant that any news fit for the paper — or not — got hand-printed on circulars, which were passed house to house. Rumor and misinformation spread with the contagion.

The awful weather did not stop Pierre from making his appointed rounds, but with the oozing mud his trips grew incomplete. "The worst roads in several years are now a certainty," reported the *Titonka Topic* on December 12. "The mud was very deep and sticky and the weather very disagreeable. A lot of rain has fallen within the past few days." These conditions meant that along with increasing demands, Pierre could not see all the patients on his list.

Mud has a starring role in an oft-told story of Sartor family dynamics. "The heaviest downpour of rain that we have ever had in Titonka and vicinity came Sunday evening," reported the local paper. "The roads and fields were a sheet of water . . . . Every cellar in the business district was flooded. . . ."

Guido's solution: They should take the car.

Pierre knew Guido loved the car and drove it well. Pierre considered their options. It was possible they would have a better chance of getting through the mud with the car rather than by taking a horse-drawn cart. *I coaxed the flivver and it started*, Guido assured him. *Easy enough to start*, Pierre retorted with some skepticism, but off they went . . . until their shiny, new Ford got stalled in thick mud beyond the edge of town. Immobilized, they waited for assistance. The time weighed heavily as Pierre fell further behind schedule. They saw the patrol wagon arrive — and pass them by. The officer had picked up a crook and had to tend to other emergencies.

With no help in sight, Pierre and Guido finally abandoned their car and began to walk home. They sloshed through deep mud in silence, trudging past one house after another. They saw neighbors' cars parked safely in their respective places. *No one else tried to drive today*, Pierre said grimly. He swore his *million thousand thunders* in French.

Guido bore his father's opprobrium in teeth-grinding silence, but when they came within sight of home, he suddenly took off, racing. In a split-second response that may have surprised them both, his middle-aged father gave chase.

Was this a good-natured sprint for father and son to blow off steam? Was Guido taunting Pierre, one-upping his *I told you so* comments about the mud and asserting himself as a near-adolescent who had to break free from his parent? Was Pierre showing that he could — literally — keep up with the son who challenged him and who got them into this difficulty, keeping Pierre from his patients? Was Pierre asserting his authority? What did he plan to do if and when he caught Guido?

We don't know, more than a century later, and it's likely they did not know then, in the heat of the moment. The ambiguity of this eruptive scene gives it dramatic power and takes us into the pressures they faced.

Then the story continues in unexpected ways . . .

Guido sprinted ahead, into the porch, and halted with a jerk just outside the front door of their home, where, remembering the family dictum not to track mud into the house, he began furiously unlacing his boots. His high leather boots were stiff, tied with a thick crisscross strap. Guido froze. He needed a buttonhook to take his boots off — but the buttonhook was inside, on his mother's dresser. All the while, Pierre was gaining on him, shouting *We never should have taken that car!* Pierre lunged into the porch just as Guido propelled himself, boots still laced, through the front door and into the house, practically cartwheeling between the furniture and his startled sisters.

Guido dashed through the house, muddy boots and all, with Pierre closing in. Guido ran into the kitchen and flung open the back door. Unfortunately, at this key moment, Guido paused again, out of habit. He grabbed the broom, as he always did, and used it to tap the screen door to scatter the pesky flies that clustered there. Doing so cost him precious time.

Then came the final blow to his plans for escape. As Pierre closed in, Guido turned, and the shoulder strap that held up his knickers got caught on a hook. There on the doorframe, he hung — and swung. Suspended, dangling, Guido pedaled his feet in midair.

By this time Mary had arrived and burst into laughter, which broke the searing tension between Pierre and Guido. It says much for her sense of humor that she enjoyed the scene and made no reproach to either of them for the muddy tracks they had splattered throughout the house. By the next week, this event was the talk of the *Titonka Topic*:

> It was evidently our doctor[']s day for hard luck, as Dr. Sartor's car died on him, south of the Dieckman place, and the doctor and son were forced to wade mud the rest of the way home.

Their neighbors enjoyed reading the newspaper report and, for years to come, Pierre and Guido would relish telling the story. They both enjoyed a good laugh, and each was the butt of this account in about equal proportion.

If we go back to the day it happened, however, there is sharp tension as the son breaks free of his father, abandoning him on a muddy street, and the father pursues his son. Everyone was teetering in those days. The flu had gone on too long. The season had been horrific, for both Pierre and Guido. And their heads were filled with nightmare stories they would like to forget.

Another car story has a more rollicking tone. It could have been a scene in one of the silent movies that played in theaters of the time. From Pierre:

> Once, Swifty Sartor was driving me to a patient. He sped through the countryside. A flock of chickens, crossing the road. Chickens usually scat but Guido was going . . . fast. I shouted: "Slow down!" We went through the flock. By the next town people pointed, laughed. We had speared a chicken on the crank handle on the lower front of the car!

Father and son turned this unexpected slaughter into a good deed. *We left the perfectly fine dead chicken with a family.* The next morning the story was news in Algona, where the motorists had made their eye-catching arrival, and for the Sartor fellows it would be a favorite memory when Guido needed a smile.

Whether by smiles or strain, Guido's world was expanding while he served Pierre as driver, companion and assistant. For other members of the Sartor family, by contrast, and their friends and neighbors, it must have seemed the walls were closing in.

Out of conviction that it was the right thing for their own health, and to set a good example for Pierre's patients and the community, Mary kept all the children except Guido at home during these weeks and months, even when others were sporadically venturing out.

Alice, the youngest daughter, would later describe how she and her siblings found ways to live around the edges of the quarantine. Their race through the garden maze, described in Chapter 1, was a favorite pursuit. Other times they would jump rope and sing on the porch, breathing in cold puffs before going back inside. But such earnest amusements could not make them forget all they were missing. Just two blocks away was Main Street . . . the French family's carriage walk . . . and the alluring aroma of fresh-baked goods at the cafe.

The shame of it was that May, who had graduated from high school in Bancroft the previous spring, and Mag, who was in high school in Titonka, were at the age when social norms called for them to prepare for marriage and motherhood. They were intelligent, accomplished and attractive, but they had no opportunity to spend time with peers at the ice cream socials, cakewalks and other occasions when youths socialized, and many fell in love.

Another Midwesterner of the era, F. Scott Fitzgerald, met his future wife, Zelda Sayre, at a country club dance that year, and made a career of writing about the ups and downs of young people's love lives. His short story "The Last of the Belles" was published in the *Saturday Evening Post* as an evocative depiction of youth who experienced romance under wartime conditions — a blend of glamor, anticipation and a sense that the world was changing around them.

Fitzgerald's description of handsome, uniformed officers and girls in fluttering gowns was a world away from what the Sartor daughters experienced during quarantine conditions in Titonka, Iowa.

Although the Sartors were a close-knit family, the children must have felt isolated, always at home. Surely, they were being cut off from their futures. May had little opportunity to socialize, so she set about writing circulars to promote women's right to vote.

Mary Sartor's dedication on the home front equaled her husband's dedication to his patients. Of course, Mary loved her children and encouraged them to pursue their interests — at one point, assisting in the cultivation of an ant farm inside a box — but aside from the races and treasure hunts she organized in the garden that adjoined their house and the children's cold-weather moments on the porch, she had very little alone time. She let some things go. She stopped using starch on laundry day to add body to the girls' dresses; just wash and rinse would do. She wasn't willing to boil the water and stir the starch. She slowed. There were days when she let young Anthony and his sisters wear their nightcaps until noon.

Mary had no outlet that was equivalent to what Pierre and Guido experienced on the road, so she sought to make one for herself at home, which prompted its own crisis with her youngest daughter.

A woman of strong faith, Mary decided she needed a chapel in their house. Her parents' home in High Ridge had a shrine, the source of much comfort to Mary when she was growing up, and the residence in Titonka had just the place: a large, second-floor landing just off the main staircase. It was perfect for Mary; but converting this space to a chapel meant dislodging Alice, who used the landing as her special play area. Alice had set up a toy ice cream parlor table and chairs in that spot, so she could play with her dolls and one favorite toy, a floppy bunny. It was also where she could get away from her sisters, who were older by four, eight and ten years. Until her mother claimed the landing, no one had noticed that Alice used it as her retreat. Eight decades later, Alice described the pain she felt at being displaced.

Alice also retained a striking visual recollection that symbolized what the family was going through that winter. Mary, according to the fashion of the era, wore a type of blouse known as a "shirtwaist." Styled after a man's dress shirt, it had buttons from waist to chin, effectively encasing the wearer. When her mother was under strain and breathing mightily, young Alice would watch the cloth loops on Mary's blouse rise and fall.

Buttoned up she may have been, but Mary could also let off steam. Bedtime brought breakdowns, and not just for children. Mary's way was to become quiet, until Pierre asked what was bothering her — a risky question. Was he oblivious to a household under quarantine with a nearly absent father and older son, while illness surged all around?

Mary had a high voice when she became undone. It would have been difficult for Pierre to listen to at the end of his own trying days. But small issues were now grown huge. This flu quarantine had put Mary off her knitting. Her priorities had been neglected too long. Mary could not go to an upcoming voice and violin recital, because no one was invited — crowds were against the rules. The sponsors could have charged 15 cents' admission, with proceeds going to the Red Cross! Any issue involving the Red Cross was important to Mary. And . . . Mayor Mousel and his wife would have their 50th wedding anniversary in Bancroft the next Sunday. Mayor Mousel, who had brought Pierre and Mary to the prairie. But did the Sartors get an invitation? No — there were no invitations — there were no gatherings during the flu. Only the couple and their priest would mark the occasion, in church. Not even Chautauqua, the traveling music show, could come through town under conditions of the flu. They brought music, dance and the arts to small towns; the Chautauqua performers raised everyone's spirits. All that was impossible now.

What was Pierre's reply to this torrent of need?

You are just going to have to get over the weeps.

To us, Pierre's reply might seem insufficient or insensitive. The fact that his words have lingered in the family's collective memory for more than a century shows their impact. At the same time, we should not judge by the standards of our generation. Despite tensions of the pandemic, the record shows Pierre and Mary were a team, which had been their consistent pattern since they left Chicago for Iowa as a young couple.

Today, we know the importance of caring for the caregiver — not only to be most effective on the job but also to protect against burnout and other risks that high-performing people face. In Pierre and Mary's time there was no discussion of concepts such as agility and resilience. We can only marvel at Pierre's coping method, expressed in his understated way, which Mary shared: *Keep on agoing.*

This exchange between Pierre and Mary, reconstructed from the family's oral tradition, also throws light on the Red Cross story in Pierre's memoir. Writing in 1953 of the "ordinary laborer" whose family was nearly destitute, Pierre praised the "special allowance of the Red Cross representative in meeting their need." When Pierre quoted himself in the account, "Tony, I send the Red Cross man down here and you get all you need," and included this event in his memoir, he must have known it would please Mary, decades after the event.

As the winter solstice approached, there were times the family was not even certain if it was night or day. Pierre and Guido left early and returned late, finding their dinner on plate warmers inside the stove, with the rest of the family in bed. When Guido fell asleep, he dreamed of what happened on their travels, blended with what he heard his father say over the telephone at home, talking to patients long into the night.

Pierre and Mary attempted some degree of normal family life. On the rare times he was home, Pierre gathered the children around. The *Titonka Topic* had a special section, "Daddy's Evening Fairy Tale," and Pierre enjoyed reading it aloud. He read to the children about nature, including grosbeaks, a beautiful songbird that May loved, and about the swallows. He used the phrase *When the swallows come* much as he told his patients *When you recover* to instill some degree of hope.

However, these cozy moments — evocative of a Norman Rockwell illustration in the *Saturday Evening Post* — were as rare as signs of spring during that bleak winter.

Pierre had another coping method, one that Guido later picked up and which is common with caregivers in many places and times. That said, it can be surprising, even shocking, to some people, including family members. This method of coping does not have an official name, but often is known as "doctor's humor" or "medical humor."

It is a fact of human psychology that devastation and crisis can lead to mirth. This may be an expression of "If you can't deal with it, laugh at it." Throughout a doctor's career and certainly for Pierre amid the pandemic, it was not possible to share details of what he saw and did during the workday — the symptoms, the tragedies — with his loved ones.

Pierre — and, from their close association, Guido — witnessed the deadly arc of influenza. Healthy in the morning, a person could be dead by midafternoon or evening.

At Saint Marys Hospital of Mayo Clinic, the Sisters of St. Francis wrote:

The disease was little understood and its vagaries were bewildering. Promising patients of whose recovery the nurses were confident, died, and 'hopeless' cases frequently recovered.

Symptoms included chills, fever, reddening and running of the nose and eyes, and dull muscular pain. Fatal cases were horrific: Patients coughed up blood and their skin color rapidly turned bluish-black. Death occurred when the patients' lungs filled with bloody sputum, causing them, in essence, to drown in their own fluids.

With scenes like this in mind, Pierre needed an alternative to answering the family's question, *What did you do today?* So, he shifted attention away from himself with stories that were humorous but also had an edge. They were typically apocryphal and featured some other, unnamed doctor — all methods of creating a safe psychological distance for Pierre and his audience. One of Pierre's stories featured a doctor whose patient had a terminal condition. The patient asked about his prognosis and the ever-diplomatic physician replied, *Well, let's just say you shouldn't begin writing a serial novel. . . .*

But no method of coping could have prepared the Sartor family for Christmas that year.

Sometimes the most important things slide when a family is overextended.

Guido had never anticipated a Christmas with more excitement, a bright light at the end of a tunnel. But into old age he would tell the sad memory of that Christmas, until we reminded him — we'd heard it. We wanted to spare him the depression; he didn't have to repeat it. Holidays can wreak havoc. For better and worse, we listened to what seemed to be Guido as a little boy, speaking to us across the years:

> *That winter . . . that Christmas morning of 1918 . . .*
> *and there was something under the tree for all, but*
> *not for me.*

His parents tried to explain . . . they didn't know how it happened . . . it had been a horrible year . . . they were so busy. But the fact was inescapable. Everyone in the family had gifts.

Only Guido was forgotten.

Perhaps it was Mother's job to arrange the gifts and Guido was mostly out of sight? He was rarely at home and Mary was done in; everyone said so. Perhaps Mary expected Pierre to get Guido's gift — after all, they spent so much time together and a father should know what his son wanted. But if that was the case, it never penetrated Pierre's awareness.

Pierre and Mary must have been in anguish. Pierre could recall the handmade gifts of his youth in Luxembourg; he and Mary had warm memories of the Christmas bounty at her elegant home in High Ridge. For the rest of their older son's life, Christmas would be tinged with a difficult memory.

Pierre tried to make amends — and succeeded only in turning a bad situation worse.

Okay, he said to Mary. *By golly, give him money.* Pierre reached into his pocket and handed Guido a fistful of cash.

Guido was working like a man, but on Christmas morning, at home with his family, he was a boy — their son. No payment for services rendered could replace a gift chosen with love.

Then the phone rang, and Pierre left to see a patient.

Tension also surfaced among the siblings. May was the oldest child and the burden of quarantine confinement must have been heavy for her — all the while seeing her younger brother go out into the world as Pierre's driver. May told their mother: *Guido got a new Boy Scout uniform; that was supposed to be for his Christmas.* A photo shows Guido in this presumptive Christmas gift, but the photo was taken the previous summer. If his big sister meant to be helpful, Guido found no solace. Decades later, however many times he told the story, he always insisted that no one ever said the uniform he received months before was intended as his Christmas gift.

Perhaps the reason Guido could never forget: The strongest memories are based in emotion. Pierre and Mary's oversight took place amid the turmoil of flu and the aftershock of war. With time, Guido could understand — but he carried this experience inside him for many years. It took place when he was 12, and the first time I heard him describe it, he was 76 years old. That never-to-be-forgotten Christmas of 1918 was the hell to be paid, when family life became trapped inside their home, with Pierre doctoring around the clock.

As the holiday season ended, Titonka settled into the lull of a prairie winter. There would be fewer social events to lure people together at this time of year under normal conditions, a fact that was intensified amid the spreading disease. People yearned for a return to normal conditions with little to show for their hopes. By the end of December, families were deep into their canned goods, stored in the pantry or on cool basement shelves. If the war made them scrape and conserve, the flu also slowed the food chain.

Food was becoming harder to come by, so they tried to preserve what they had. Grapes were stored in bran, eggs in lime water. They used Knox's Sparkling Calves Foot Gelatin to make the food they had stretch further.

To avoid face-to-face contact, customers left coins in a shoebox on the porch, where farmers could drop off goods and pick up their payment. For the most part, the honor system worked, but by isolating people from one another, the social fabric became frayed.

Life at home for the people of Titonka had been the same for a very long time, made worse in the relentless dark of shortened winter days. Everyone was in the capsule of their own little world: Neverland . . . in bungalows.

Tensions and pressures facing the Sartor family did not abate. After the holidays came another encounter, still vivid after more than a century, which uneasily combines a father's frustration and his son's sense of wonder. It does not take a psychiatrist to see that this story, as well as the muddy chase, features Pierre and Guido bursting out of the confines of their environment.

Pierre and Guido were on the road days into nights, with moist cold winds blowing upon them. One night, home at last, Pierre huddled in the kitchen, the fire out, while Guido slumped into bed. Pierre was so tired that his eyes felt parched in their sockets. Adding misery to exhaustion, he had contracted dry heaves from one of his patients, a woman with the flu. He cleaned her, then himself, soiled from close contact with his patient, and within hours the doctor was ill.

Now, before the day was done, he needed boiling water to sanitize his medical instruments. Out of habit — and it is telling that Pierre was so stressed and exhausted that he did not realize he was in his own house — he called for his nurse. Of course, no nurse came. So, he boiled the water himself, but it was a struggle. His dry eyes squinted and blinked. Pierre waited impatiently, willed himself to stay awake. But as the water reached a rolling boil, something inside him cracked.

Pierre seized the pan — if it was cast iron, typical for the time, it would have been hot and heavy with water gurgling and popping — and made straight for the back door. What was he thinking? Did he imagine himself heading to a patient, water sloshing? Or had he reached his breaking point, just as the water started to boil?

Guido must have heard Pierre's steps. Always in tow to his father, he got out of bed and followed Pierre in a reverse of their mud-spattered pursuit through the house.

The air was dry that frigid night, and Pierre went out behind a snowbank. Guido followed in silence. With a vigorous thrust, Pierre threw the boiling water high into the air, his arm making an arc. Out of the pan water flew and froze, suspended and sparkling, lit by the moon and stars. It was only a moment, but the magic seemed much longer, until the water turned into tiny ice pellets and showered down.

We don't know exactly when Pierre realized that Guido was with him. Did Pierre toss the boiling water in savage frustration while Guido, unbeknownst to his father, stood back and watched? Pierre would long describe this night as the time he broke. Or did Pierre set out from the kitchen in confusion and frustration, only to perceive Guido following him and, seizing the moment with a wink in his eye, create a delightful scene his son would always remember?

Pierre and Guido were together in a snow globe of their own making. *Do it again!* Guido begged in this moment between youth and adulthood. But it could not be repeated.

The new year brought a resolution that broke Guido's heart.

Pierre replaced Guido as his driver with a man named Bill Senne, a neighbor.

Pierre's reasoning is not known, although several factors were likely involved. The flu was still rampant, but there was a growing sense in Titonka and elsewhere — which Pierre must have known and perhaps accepted — that influenza could not be completely prevented, much less eradicated. People would have to learn to live with it. Pierre's plan of sanitation and isolation made sense, especially for affected families, but life had to go on. The schools would reopen eventually and in an agricultural society like Titonka, everyone knew that the farmers — and their children, helping — would have to put in the crops according to nature's schedule, influenza or not. It was time for Guido to return to the rhythms of ordinary life, insofar as that was possible.

By January 1919, Pierre had been fighting influenza, with ever-greater intensity, patient volumes and geographic reach, for more than three months. He must have prayed nightly that he and his son would not get ill, so they could continue the work that was set before them. He must have found strength that, in the words of St. Francis of Assisi, he was doing "what was mine to do." But Pierre could not involve Guido in this medical mission for the long term, especially when his hopes for Guido required that he undertake years of education.

As the driver, Guido had met an immediate, pressing need, but Pierre's view of the situation was changing. He was moving beyond crisis response to a long-term effort. This is another example of the systems thinking that aligned with the Mayo brothers. However, while a systems methodology supports making changes that are justified by empirical evidence, which was certainly the case as Pierre surveyed his need for transportation in the foreseeable future, change can come at a human cost. That cost is especially high when it is borne within a family — and by a son who honors his father.

Pierre had good reasons to contact Bill Senne for the job. In his roughly 60-year medical practice, Pierre had many colleagues and friends, but he never valued any of them more than he did the likes of Bill Senne, the kind of person always willing to roll up his sleeves and take on the work that needed to be done. Bill was solid and dependable, but their road trips would be quite different from when Pierre and his son were a team.

Another change came to Pierre's plan. Rather than return home, however late, at the end of his rounds, he now tended to stay overnight with his patients. This may indicate that Pierre was able to provide more time and effort to a diminishing number of people with influenza.

It also meant that Dr. Sartor and neighbor Bill Senne would not have the regular togetherness that father and son experienced, departing each morning for a full day's work. On top of that, Bill was a self-sufficient adult with a life of his own; he could not be at Pierre's beck and call, ready to devote long hours to assist Pierre. One can forgive Guido if he felt perhaps a rueful satisfaction that his replacement, the much-praised Bill Senne, wound up being only an occasional help to his father, after all.

We do not know if Pierre realized Bill Senne would be unable to provide the ongoing service he needed . . . if Bill stepped back and qualified what assistance he could offer . . . or if Guido stepped forward, making clear his availability and willingness . . . but at some point Guido returned to the driver's seat, at least part of the time.

He was there for what became, in many respects, their longest and most meaningful journey together.

This brings us back to the event that began our story.

When Pierre and Guido set off that day, they were reunited as physician and driver and, despite their recent friction, as father and son. This particular trip involved taking two horse-drawn vehicles and a railroad handcar to reach their destination; the family's Ford motorcar, which featured in so many recent adventures, was parked safely at home.

It was just after Groundhog Day, a time when many people

on the prairie dare to hope for spring, even with scant evidence in sight. For the people of Titonka, however, Groundhog Day 1919 seemed to take the weather backward. After a winter of mud and temperatures in the 30s and 40s, Titonka was now in the grip of a cold snap. *Mother Earth white with snow . . . The snow piled several feet in some places.*

Conditions would get far worse before Pierre and Guido made it back home.

It had been four months since influenza arrived aboard the Klondike train on October 1 of the previous year. Since then, Pierre had gained valuable experience treating influenza and its attendant scourge, pneumonia. He had researched, developed and modified his plan according to the needs and opportunities that arose, and had seen his plan prove its validity.

Pierre did not know it on that morning, but he had approximately six weeks left before the disease would begin to run its course and eventually dissipate. In his 1953 memoir, written when he had the perspective to analyze his experience, Pierre calculated that his practice during the influenza pandemic spanned from early October 1918 through mid-March 1919, although in other locations it lasted longer. During that time, he provided care to more than 1,100 bedridden patients — along with a larger number of "perambulatory cases" — and, throughout that time, he lost only five patients.

Well before any official reckoning of data from fatalities in the state, nation and world, Pierre knew that his record compared favorably to other practitioners'. Pierre's medical school classmate, Dr. James Dill Robertson, as health commissioner for the city of Chicago, had presided over more than 2,000 cases from influenza and pneumonia per day during the previous October.

Adding to the pressure, caregivers in nearby towns were becoming ill and dying. Some were volunteers while others, such as Dr. Dolmage's nurse, were medical professionals. Woden was under the care of Dr. Ray. When he became ill, Pierre took over Dr. Ray's territory, extending the area where Pierre had to travel and serve.

This meant that Pierre was starting over again, advocating for sanitation and isolation, building a network of volunteers to assist in caring for patients and providing shelter for their families. House to house, farm to farm, they went, Pierre and Guido, leaving written directions.

The story that began this book is the last account in Pierre's memoir. As with his other case reports, it combines human interest and medical information, and demonstrates the interweaving of human relationships. It comes immediately after the Red Cross story that must have warmed Mary Sartor's heart.

> *Not far from this place a mother came down with the flu and a severe pneumonia complication. A little daughter about 4 years old was the next case. In a little bed at the opposite corner of the room.*

We can piece together that Pierre called upon this mother and child several times and arranged for volunteer help from the wife of Tony, the "attendant man" who had secured items from the Red Cross for the laborer's family. We do not know the last name of Tony and his wife or the circumstances of their lives, but they must have been a remarkable couple, devoting themselves to the care of others and working in trusted collaboration with Dr. Sartor. Pierre wrote: "The mother improved, some owing to the good care of Tony's wife (the one who took care of the buggy case)."

Pierre's ability to establish relationships with his patients — on a personal as well as a professional basis — is on display in the sickroom conversation that he described: "Mother looked at me and said, pointing to the little girl, 'Doctor, if you make that one well again, you can ask of me anything you wish for.'"

As with most of his patients, Pierre knew the mother had little in the way of financial means. But from the time and effort he invested in her care, he knew her as a person, and he knew she had a special quality: "The mother was a good singer."

Pierre did not practice medicine for the money he could make. Financial reward would never be the motivation for why he worked this long, this hard, in this particularly grim winter. He was well past his youthful quest for status.

Instead, Pierre had found far better compensation by getting to know his patients — medically, personally and even spiritually. As Dr. Charles H. Mayo wrote, "Medicine gives only to those who give, but her reward for those who serve is 'finer than much fine gold.'"

In this moment, coming after the grueling trip that he and Guido took just to reach this patient, Pierre deflected the topic of finances. On the spot, he came up with terms that show his heart as a caregiver: "'All right,' I said, 'I want you and your daughter some day to sing for me.'"

Pierre handled the situation with tact. In addition to providing medical service and coordinating follow-up care from Tony's wife, Pierre found a way to show respect for his patient without the burden of financial obligation.

It was not the first or last time Pierre evinced such deftness in a patient relationship. But this encounter proved to be different.

It took place on February 3, the day after Groundhog Day, but Pierre would come to describe the date as April Fools' Day. Without realizing it, he had set in motion one of the great surprises of his life — although it would take many years before Pierre received his payment.

As Pierre struggled with the demands of caring for patients during the influenza pandemic and saw the toll it took upon his own family, he turned to the comforting words of the Physician's Prayer.

A Physician's Prayer

Dear Lord, Thou Great Physician, I kneel before Thee. Since every good and perfect gift must come from

Thee I pray;

Give skill to my hand, clear vision to my mind, kindness and sympathy to my heart. Give me singleness of purpose, strength to lift at least a part of the burden of my suffering fellowmen and a true realization of the privilege that is mine. Take from my heart all guile and worldliness that with the simplest faith of a child I may rely on Thee. Amen.

Litho in U.S.A.   H-N.Y.   E-43

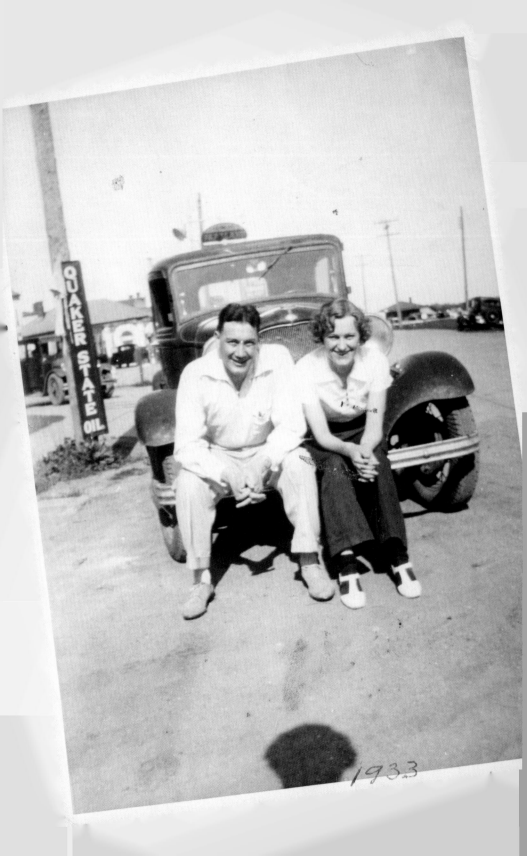

1933

CHAPTER 19

"Doing nicely"

Titonka, Iowa
1919-1945

"ABOUT A YEAR AFTER THE EPIDEMIC I read in a medical paper that in some flu camps in the South 'isolation' was practiced, a tent for each patient and the result was wonderful."

Even in the midst of fighting influenza, Pierre knew his methods of isolation worked. This reference in his memoir provides additional validation. The paper that Pierre read and referred to was part of the medical profession's widespread assessment of treatment methods following the pandemic.

Mayo Clinic joined this effort when Dr. William J. Mayo commissioned a study of best practices in hospital design, which was published in 1919 as an article entitled "The Organization and Methods of Contagious Disease Services" by Dr. John H. Stokes, a member of the staff of Mayo Clinic. This study involved research and benchmarking at Mayo and other leading medical centers. The results were published and presented to

The author's parents, Dr. Guido and Luella Sartor. Pierre said Luella was "the best thing that ever happened" to his son — words that Luella cherished all her life.

community-based medical societies throughout the United States, showing the wide applicability of its findings. Looking to the future, the study concluded:

If professional knowledge is quick to take advantage of an aroused public interest, a new cooperation between physician and layman will bring about advances comparable to those which war has stimulated in other fields of medical practice.

Findings from Mayo's research, therefore, aligned with Pierre's insistence upon isolation and the collaborative network of volunteers he established to help care for patients and provide shelter for their families.

What he accomplished in serving patients and saving lives was a source of personal and professional satisfaction to Pierre. But for a man who entitled his memoir "Thrills of my life — specifically my 'Flu Life,'" the question arose as to what would happen once the crisis had passed.

Pierre used the analogy of a prairie wildfire to describe the rapid spread of influenza, and his comparison is equally true for how the pandemic ended. The influenza of 1918-1919, in essence, extinguished itself. Intense and widespread, it claimed the lives of the most vulnerable patients and created "herd immunity" by infecting many other people who survived. By 1919-1920, it became much more difficult for the virus to find new people to infect. This, in turn, sharply curtailed its ability to reproduce and spread.

But as outbreaks of influenza diminished, the effects of the disease persisted. As the State Historical Society of Iowa concluded: "Thus, the epidemic's impact was felt for years after the crisis ended, both in social terms and with respect to the physical aftereffects — including weakening of the heart, lungs, liver and kidneys — experienced by the flu's victims."

Pierre had saved many lives in Titonka and the surrounding area during the pandemic. It is likely that his post-influenza practice included care for flu survivors who dealt with long-term consequences of the disease. The lingering, tragic reach of the pandemic came home to Pierre and Mary when her brother, Alfred (Freddie) Winandy, died on July 2, 1919, from complications of the influenza he had contracted months before. The *Titonka Topic* reviewed Freddie's life over the past year, stating that he "underwent a severe attack of the flu, which left him in weakened condition, and he never fully recovered."

Even without the pandemic, there was plenty to keep Pierre active in his small-town, rural practice, as seen in these examples from the spring of 1920:

> *Fred Boyken stepped on a rusty nail Monday morning which protruded nearly two inches into his foot. Dr. Sartor dressed the wound and he is reported doing nicely.*

> *Albert Meyer . . . expects to go into the chicken business extensively this year and has selected a good location for the industry. [He installed a manure carrier as part of his business and] had the misfortune to catch one of his fingers, inflicting a painful as well as serious wound, and it was thought for a time that he might lose the finger. Dr. Sartor was called and the wound is doing nicely at this time.*

As these quotations indicate, "doing nicely" was a frequent description of Pierre's patients in this era. The chatty coverage of his medical services shows Pierre as professionally capable and highly respected.

> *W.H. Stott, our neighbor, while fixing a pump Monday, accidentally tore the nail off one of his thumbs. When he arrived at the office of Dr. Sartor he fainted and fell on the floor. When [he] regained consciousness the Dr. was pummeling him with his fists to start the circulation and heart to beating.*

Pierre might not have used the word "thrills" from his memoir to describe it, but a new, satisfying avenue of activities opened for him at this time. After the war and pandemic, he could pursue civic activities that had not been possible when he first moved to Titonka. Pierre joined the Lions Club. A friend recalled: "My first acquaintance with Dr. Sartor came at the

Three Winandy Sisters

Susan Jacquer

Mary Sartor

Regina
Winandy

Titonka Lions Club where I heard the roar of his hearty laughter above that of all the others."

In civic matters, Pierre served on the Water Board of the City Council and was president of the Chamber of Commerce. He helped lead the successful effort to install a storm and sanitation system, which a fellow council member described as "a large order for a small town." In addition:

> The climax of our being together on the Council came when we felt it was time to put in a City water System. This had been tried a number of times previously but had failed; we succeeded, however. . . . Dr. Sartor was as much of a success as a Council Man as our doctor here in Titonka.

Mary had some health problems in the postwar era that caused her to slow down. Fortunately, they did not stop her enjoyment of family and community and activities. She continued with her church and civic pursuits. Newspaper accounts describe her as an active member and diligent officer of the Titonka Women's Club, hosting meetings and presenting on topics such as South American Opera, The National Art Gallery, Keeping Up with Medicine, and Our Right to Live, Our Concern for Other People's Welfare and Handicapped Children.

Pierre and Mary's daughters were growing up. As stated in an article about Pierre in the *Des Moines Tribune*: "His family has followed his example of community service." May became a primary school teacher; Magdalene was a teacher in the area around Titonka; Mercedes became a nurse in Chicago; Alice earned a degree in podiatry in Chicago and practiced in Charles City, Iowa.

Regarding both their sons, Pierre and Mary felt concern.

Anthony was becoming more and more delicate. By December 1926, when Anthony was 12 years old, he began to decline

After the influenza crisis, Mary (center) resumed her frequent travels to visit family and friends. Here she joined her sisters Susan (formally known as Susanna, left) and Regina (right).

and never returned to school. At night he was bedridden; during the day, if the weather was fine and he was able, he was taken outside to sit in the sunshine, using a wheelchair.

Pierre's heart churned into what felt like a figure eight. He was a doctor and could not cure his son. Was he at fault? Pierre's father, Mathias, with less education and fewer resources, had made it possible for Pierre's childhood hearing problem to be treated. Yet now, after medical science had made great progress and he had established a successful practice, Pierre had no answers for his son's decline.

And then . . . Guido. His high school years were a time of accomplishment and excitement. During the summer of 1920, he repeated the wartime journey he made with Mary and, as he wrote for his grandchildren, "drove 400 miles to Chicago when 14 as the only driver."

Around the same time, Guido developed a new hobby, embracing the latest communications technology. "Fred Thomas, a garage mechanic who also knew electronics, encouraged me to get a radio license and build my own radio station. My radio station reached Russia and the Philippines and Melbourne, Australia, by the time I was sixteen."

In 1923, Guido graduated as valedictorian of his class, not yet 17 years old. Pierre was so proud. From 1923 to 1925, Guido attended Columbia College (today, Loras College) in Dubuque, Iowa, where he was a member of the men's choir. He also pursued his radio hobby, notwithstanding the fact that it was against college rules.

One day Guido had an antenna hanging out his dorm window as a priest walked by beneath. It is said that as he hastily pulled in the antenna, it crashed to the pavement below . . . and it is not known what happened next!

Electronics were a passion for Guido his entire life. When he and my mother were finally able to build the house they wanted, Daddy splurged on a top-of-the-line Scott radio. My mother's eyes glittered. *That radio*, she said, *costs as much as a car!* I understand Mom's feelings, but it was Daddy's love of tape recorders and the like that got Pierre to record his memories.

Guido enrolled at the University of Iowa in 1926 and took a variety of summer courses and correspondence work. He expressed the desire to go into medicine, following his father's example. But for a variety of reasons — likely including the lack of money — his educational journey stalled.

Along with Anthony's frail health, the financial constraints upon Guido were a burden for Pierre — another reason for him to feel inadequate. Back in Luxembourg, Mathias Sartor had seen to Pierre's education, which had opened a lifetime of opportunities. Pierre could not do the same for his elder son. For years, Pierre had been willing to receive chickens and produce as payment for his medical services, and he would continue this practice throughout his career. G.D. Hart, a civil engineer in Bancroft, who knew Pierre, wrote: "The good doctor has never become wealthy due, perhaps, to the fact that his skills in collecting his service fee is far inferior to his skill as a mender of ailing human bodies and faltering souls." Pierre's noble philosophy meant he could not fund the dream of medical school that he and Guido shared.

After Columbia College, Guido taught in the country schools around Titonka. A newspaper article published years later included a photo of Guido from 1927 in sporty attire with a description of how he boarded with a local family when he taught school. The article says Guido:

> recalls the social life of the community, the card parties, the game parties and also dancing parties in various homes. He states that, being of Luxembourg background, he enjoyed teaching children who, when excited, spoke [the dialect of] Luxembourg, thus putting the books on the "schaf" as often as in the bookcase.

I think this must have amused Guido because "schaf" (meaning "shelf") was one of the Luxembourg words he learned at the age of 11 on his visit to Grandfather Winandy in Chicago during the summer of 1917.

Guido was a grown man by now, but father and son still managed to find themselves in automobile adventures on the winter roads:

> Dr. Sartor started to take his son Guido to his school
> at St. Joe on Sunday and when south of Algona a few
> miles, something about the car broke down and the
> Dr. and the schoolmaster were left setting out in the
> ten below zero weather. He called Otto Falk of the
> Falk Motor Co., who drove down and took Guido on
> to his school and pulled the Dr. and his Ford coupe
> home. It was a cold and fast ride for the Dr. on his
> return trip.

After teaching during the academic year, Guido spent summers in Chicago, working in greenhouse construction for his grandfather's business. The booming stock market of the 1920s made greenhouses a popular home improvement for many well-to-do families. After several summers in Chicago, Guido branched out and went to work for Frank Murphy, one of his grandfather's friends who also had a greenhouse company. This entailed a move to Urbana, Ohio.

Summers with the Murphys seemed glamorous to Guido. He knew he was special to Frank and his wife, Mamie. Guido slipped easily into their social scene, and into the setting of beautiful homes and cars and a circle of sophisticated young friends. It was a Midwestern version of what F. Scott Fitzgerald described in his novel *The Great Gatsby*: "In his blue gardens men and girls came and went like moths among the whisperings and the champagne and the stars."

In the fall of 1927, Guido returned to Titonka. Anthony needed more help than his parents could give. Guido, a caregiver at heart with a strong commitment to his family, decided to move back home so he could assist with Anthony.

It was during that year that Guido began dating Luella Recker. A dance in Lakota, Iowa, brought them together. Guido danced with Luella every time he could get his name onto her dance card. At the end of the evening, he asked to take her home. But Luella's mother had a rule: *If you can get to a dance, you can come home the same way.* Luella had to say no.

From then on, Guido arranged for the two of them to ride

along with Luella's sister Leone and her future husband, Lermond Intermill, who had a car. One day Guido would say his fondest memory of "sparking," as dating was called at the time, was to ride home in Lermond's rumble seat with Luella on his lap.

Guido and Luella had known each other since their elementary school days in Bancroft. Now they laughed and reminisced about how their paths had crossed years before, when his family and hers were in the automobile showroom on the same day.

Sometimes they went to dances in a Lakota theater that featured well-known orchestras. When it became too warm, they moved to Woods Lake, an open pavilion. Also in the summer, they went to dances at the Hands Park and Interlaken summer resorts.

In the fall, Luella resumed her work as a teacher in a country school. Almost every day when school let out, Guido was there to meet Luella. In the winter, they went to dances: Wednesday evenings in Bancroft and Friday evenings in Titonka.

Soon Pierre and Mary could see that Guido and Luella were in love.

One day, over seven decades later, Guido, then in his 90s, returned to Buffalo Center, where Luella had grown up, to visit what he called his "old stomping grounds." Guido's son-in-law David Beckman videotaped the walk. Arriving at the farmhouse where Luella's family had lived, Guido pointed to an enormous oak tree. Elderly, emotional, he recounted the moment: *I kissed Luella for the first time under that tree — and the tree is still standing!*

On May 25, 1928, Anthony turned 14. Pierre said it was time to have a professional photo taken of Anthony wearing a man's suit. He was past the age when boys wore knickers. Was Pierre remembering his own father, Mathias, who arranged a photo of Pierre about the same age, when Pierre's health was as uncertain as Anthony's?

Pierre, Guido and Anthony drove to Winona, Minnesota, to the Van Vranken Studio where Guido had been photographed almost a decade before, when he was 13. It is a sign of the family's frugality that Anthony wore the same suit that Guido had worn in his portrait. Pierre and Guido helped Anthony out of the car and carried him to a spot by a tree.

The brothers looked so alike that years later one member of the family mailed a copy of the picture to a relative and wrote an inscription on the back, identifying the young man in the photo as Guido. But the photo is of Anthony. In another print taken that day, 22-year-old Guido can be seen in the background, standing next to a wheelchair, its large wheels and curved grip bars making a somber silhouette against the sky.

With the coming of summer, Guido prepared to return to Ohio. Luella kept Guido's letters, which today are part of the family archive. One is dated June 1928:

> Hi Luella Dearest:
> I cannot help but realize that this is the last nite. (Till when?) When will we meet again? What does Dewey do on a dew-dew-dewey day? Where does Lermond's moustache go when he laughs?

A few more lines of poetry, not Guido's, and he closed the letter with polite formality:

> I'll meet you again next spring. Guido J. Sartor

Guido could make no promises. He might stay in Ohio for the next year and go into construction. There were hints of another promotion.

Would Luella be there when he returned? Pierre remembered himself at Guido's age when he left Mary to investigate Iowa.

Guido knew that other boys would want to date Luella. She was a good dancer and a lot of fun, a pretty blonde with a tiny waist and big blue eyes. She was also a determined young woman. In order to attend the town high school in Buffalo

Pierre and Mary's youngest son, Anthony, proudly wore a man's suit for this photo. He was frail — note his wheelchair in the background — and died in 1929, shortly after his 15th birthday.

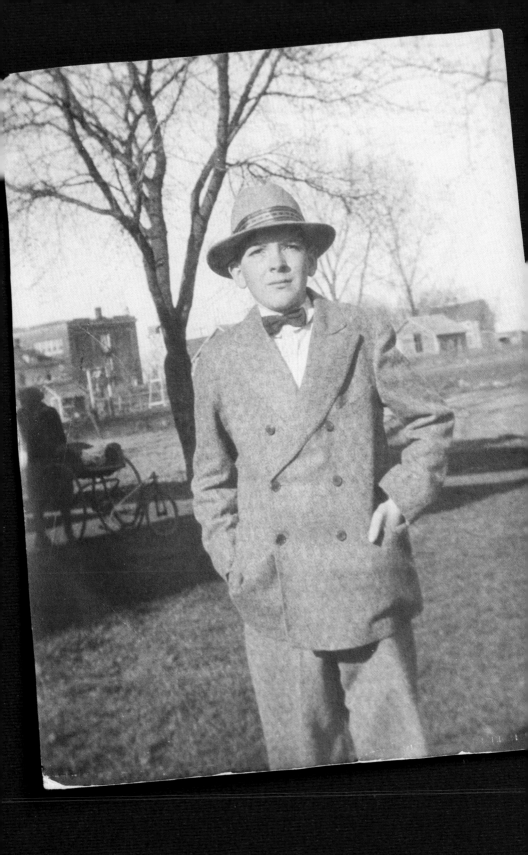

Center, she had walked six miles round trip from her family's farm each day. When she decided she wanted to be a violinist in the school orchestra, she taught herself to play. Like Guido, she was the valedictorian of her class.

As Guido was making plans to head back to Ohio, Pierre learned from his network of patients and friends that Luella and Leone had been invited to a nearby farm to teach a Methodist woman's sons to dance. Dance was against the family's religion, but the mother thought it was important they learn how in that era of the Charleston and fox trot, and she figured that no one needed to know — although word got around to Pierre.

The Recker girls were popular. Toward the end of her life, Luella wrote a memoir that she entitled *Life in the Fast Lane*. As she described: "We did have good times at those parties … Would you believe all three of those boys got to be good dancers and we always remained good friends?"

Before Guido left for Ohio, he told his father that one day, he hoped to marry Luella. But he felt he should be more settled before he proposed.

Pierre remembered how it felt to find a woman who was beautiful, intelligent and willing to do what it took to live her dream. He hoped that things would work out for Guido and Luella. Pierre had an additional measure of respect for Luella: Her father, Henry, had left home at age 15, with his 17-year-old brother, Joseph, to make their place in the world. Initiative and hard work were part of Luella's character.

For Guido, his return to Ohio was much the same as before, filled with parties and glamour. His friendship with Mr. and Mrs. Murphy deepened. They even said they would like to adopt Guido. But as he explained, "I already have a family."

In the spring of 1929, Guido returned to Titonka. Anthony had become so ill that he was admitted to St. Joseph Hospital in Mankato, Minnesota, which decades later would become part of Mayo Clinic Health System. In April, a blizzard blanketed the region. Guido took photos of Luella standing on her tiptoes, reaching for the top of a snowbank.

The schools were closed due to the spring blizzard. Guido could now see Luella any day he could get through the snow. Strong with determination, he made numerous trips to see her, notwithstanding the snow-packed roads.

In early June, Anthony returned home from the hospital. Heart disease was making him progressively weaker. We have wondered within the family if Pierre consulted his colleagues at Mayo Clinic or at Loyola University, successor to his medical school in Chicago, for advice about helping Anthony. There is no concrete information, but it would have made sense for Pierre to do so.

Anthony faced his future with grace, which inspired those around him. I am sure he and Guido drew comfort from a framed text of The Twelve Promises of the Sacred Heart of Jesus in the bedroom they shared.

The weeks in Titonka went by. Anxious friends hovered by Anthony's bed. Pierre and Mary were moved by their understanding and love. Their sensitivity touched Pierre deeply.

The *Titonka Topic* praised Anthony's

> *... many fine qualities and especially ... the charity of his words and thoughts for those less fortunate than he. He always had a kind word for everyone. He was a deeply religious boy and during his suffering was sustained and comforted by it.*
>
> *... With an unusually active mind and keen wit, Anthony, although physically handicapped, took a great interest in the happenings of the world in which he lived. He was a great reader and conversation with him displayed a wide range of interest and knowledge far beyond his years. During all the months of his illness we have visited him often and never have found him to be self-pitying ... because of his infirmity. He enjoyed his family and his friends and was touchingly grateful for every thought and act which contributed to his comfort and welfare.*

Pierre expressed gratitude to everyone who reached out to Anthony at this time. What Pierre did not say aloud, but which

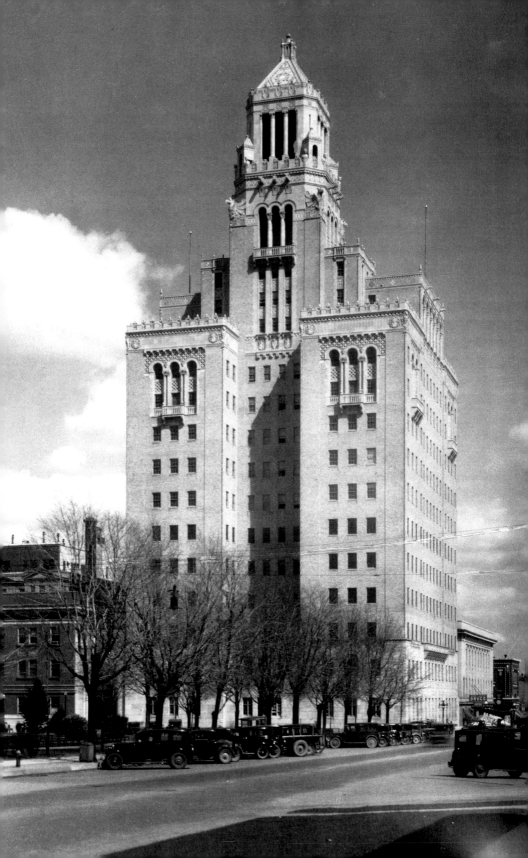

he certainly felt, was *My heart break.*

In 1996, family members filmed a video of Guido returning to his old home in Titonka. The camera followed him as he entered the main-floor bedroom that he had shared with Anthony when they were boys. Guido was surprised and deeply touched to see a framed print on the wall — The Twelve Promises of the Sacred Heart of Jesus — just as it had been there when he and Anthony were young, when both of them read it with devotion as the younger brother's health declined.

Anthony Reginald Henry Sartor died on September 30, 1929. He was just four months past his 15th birthday.

In deepest grief, Pierre turned to his surviving son, who had struggles of his own. Guido was casting about; his cherished days of caring for Anthony were now over. With Anthony gone, both Pierre and Guido lost a driving force in their lives. Mary Sartor and Guido's sisters shared in the sorrow.

Soon the family had to say goodbye to Guido. And Guido said goodbye to Luella. Resolutely facing his future, he drove to Ohio and paid a call on Frank and Mamie Murphy at their beautiful home. They listened to the sad story of Anthony's death. They had lost a son of their own and could empathize all too well. The Murphys extended a heartfelt welcome to Guido.

As before, Guido worked for the Murphys and plunged into a whirlwind of social events. Photos show Guido and friends in swimsuits, lined up by the running board of a sports car. There were picnics in the garden and dances in the pavilion, with young people lounging in the gazebo. Mamie Murphy loved to entertain.

And then came "the fairy story, the miracle of our lives," as Luella would write one day.

Even Pierre, who had sought a miracle for his health and his

When Guido drove his mother to Mayo Clinic in 1930, they saw Mayo's new diagnostic building. Guido was already thinking about a career in medicine.

mother's while he was a boy in Luxembourg, was taken aback by this change of fortune.

One evening, Mr. and Mrs. Murphy invited Guido into their sun porch. Under the shimmering glass, with a view of the manicured gardens that Guido had once tended, they told him that they had grown to love him, almost from the start. Guido, they said, had become the son they had lost so long ago.

On that day, at sunset, Frank Murphy asked Guido: *What do you really want to do with your life?* With Guido's slender build and long, delicate hands, Mr. Murphy did not see him continuing to work in construction.

Guido later said he had no idea what the couple had in mind.

He answered them, simply: *I would like to be a doctor, like my father.*

Frank and Mamie Murphy then extended an offer Guido could scarcely believe: to put him through medical school, tuition and board.

Guido returned home with the wonderful news. To Pierre, it seemed his life had come full circle. Decades before, Pierre's brothers had funded his medical education. Now, Frank and Mamie Murphy were providing the same support to his son.

At this time, Guido formed his own connection with Mayo Clinic. It lasted throughout his career and into retirement. As the *Kossuth County Advance* noted on August 24, 1930:

> *Mrs. Pierre Sartor and son Guido drove to Rochester, Minn., last week Thursday, where Mrs. Sartor went through the Mayo clinic.*

Less than two years before Guido and Mary arrived in Rochester, Mayo Clinic had opened a 15-story building, which remains a focal point of Mayo's campus today. We can imagine the inspiration Guido felt at this early stage of his medical studies when he took in the building's ornate architectural

Guido (right) met Frank and Mamie Murphy when he worked for their greenhouse construction firm. Having lost a son years before, the Murphys bonded with Guido and sponsored his medical education.

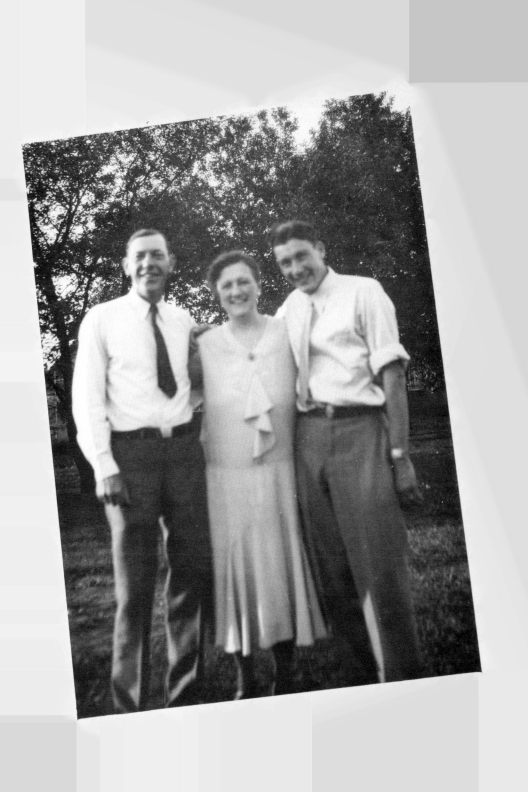

details, massive bronze doors at the entrance and bell tower that crowned the structure, along with its efficient systems to serve thousands of patients.

There was another dimension to these exciting times: Following his father's footsteps, with medicine confirmed as his career, Guido was ready to get married.

Pierre told Luella she was the best thing that ever happened to Guido. Those words meant the world to my mother — that day and for the rest of her life.

As a courtesy to Mr. and Mrs. Murphy, Guido asked if getting married would change their arrangement. Mamie Murphy assured him that funds for tuition and board would continue as planned. Medical school proved to be an ideal focus for Guido's intelligence and commitment. At the end of his first year, he received a commendation from the dean of the medical school for his standing as fifth in a class of 125 students. He served as vice president of the campus chapter of Alpha Kappa Kappa, a medical fraternity, in his junior year.

Guido's transformative experience parallels that of Charles W. (Chuck) Mayo, who, like Guido, was the son of a highly regarded physician, Charles H. Mayo. Chuck also struggled in school and later wrote: "It wasn't surprising that as a young man I should have a wretched sense of my own inferiority." Chuck's crisis was to develop rheumatic fever while in college. He recovered at the home of family friends who, as Mr. and Mrs. Murphy did with Guido, gave him perspective and purpose. Chuck wrote that they "healed the sense of aching inadequacy that I had been feeling ever since my boyhood. . . . I gained a sense of my own worth and the courage to believe in it."

Guido needed to draw on those reserves of self-confidence because the first years of his marriage, during the grim years of the early 1930s, were a challenge. Guido and Luella lived in Iowa City on the allotment that Mr. and Mrs. Murphy provided, as best they could, for a while. One day Luella would reflect: "It is true that two can live as cheaply as one — only if one isn't hungry."

Their life echoed the lyrics of "My Blue Heaven," a popular song of the era — "Molly and me, and baby makes three." Celeste Marie Donna Jean Sartor was born on June 4, 1932. Luella returned to Titonka, staying with Pierre and Mary, toward the end of her pregnancy. To make Luella feel welcome, Pierre had a little joke. He said that since he had delivered Luella's sister, Leone, it was now time to claim Luella. He and Mary were delighted to help in any way.

Guido came to Titonka over his summer break, and the three of them lived above Pierre's office. The time passed quickly, until Guido had to return to his studies. Reluctantly, they decided that Luella and Celeste should stay and live with Luella's family on their farm near Buffalo Center.

As Luella would one day write:

> It was very difficult for me to stay behind with the baby when Guido went back to school. It was the only way that we could make it and I was lucky that I could stay at home, on the farm with my parents and brothers and sister, outside of Buffalo Center. It wasn't easy for students to be married while in college at the time. Of course, our struggles occurred when most people were dealing with the Depression. The farm was the best place for the two of us [mother and daughter] to be — we always had plenty to eat. I had good training from my mother on how to get along, make do and do without and still be happy.

Luella brought Celeste to visit Guido periodically, and one summer joined him on a trip to Ohio to meet Frank and Mamie Murphy. But these visits were short. As he immersed himself in medical studies, Guido brought home with him the smell of formaldehyde, a pungent experience for mother and child, especially in warm weather before the invention of air conditioning.

The family had cause for celebration when Guido received his Doctor of Medicine degree on June 1, 1936, ranked 11th in a class of 96 graduates. Celeste, a toddler by then, made the ceremony memorable when she stood up on the riser and shouted,

That's my daddy!

Medicine had become far more specialized since Pierre's graduation and Guido sought opportunities for advanced training. He was accepted to a residency at the University of Chicago. Again, complications intervened. Guido planned to study surgery, but he developed Dupuytren's contracture, a hand deformity that affects tissue under the skin of the palm. Knots of tissue create a thick cord that pulls one or more fingers into a bent position. This interferes with daily activities such as putting on gloves or shaking hands, and, even after Guido had an operation, it meant that surgery would not be the career path he would follow.

As Pierre often said: *Nothing easy.*

Guido switched to pediatrics, but this meant he had to extend his time in residency. Adding to the burden was continued separation from his family. Luella and Celeste joined him in Chicago for a time but, again, three living in a small room was difficult. Luella took Celeste back to Iowa.

When Celeste reached school age, Luella moved from her family's farm to the nearby community of Buffalo Center and went to work for her brother, Chuck, who owned a movie theater. A skilled seamstress, Luella sewed a pants uniform for herself and then made a few more pairs for everyday use, thus becoming the first woman in Buffalo Center to wear trousers.

Luella also earned money by taking in men's suits to restyle for women; by cutting off the worn knees, she made trousers into skirts. Her skills met a need for thrifty families in those years of economic hardship, and the orders poured in. She sold about 100 refashioned suits to women in Buffalo Center and the surrounding communities, charging $3 each. Guido figured those suits must have been seen on women walking up and down the main streets of those little towns — half a dozen at any given time!

Now in his 60s, Pierre remained in practice while Guido was establishing himself in the medical profession. The Great Depression began with the stock market crash in New York City but soon extended its grip across the country, including the activities of the Kossuth County Medical Society:

> *An all-time low was hit in January, 1934, when Dr. Sartor, the secretary, recorded transactions at a meeting where "six members were present, and there were no subjects, no discussion, no papers and no plans. Meeting adjourned sine die" [indefinitely, with no set date for resumption].*

Hard times limited Pierre's income but not the level of service he provided to patients. In February 1936, as described in the *Titonka Topic*, he put technology and ingenuity to work, along with his well-established ability to work with volunteers:

> *Mr. and Mrs. Jesse Harms are the parents of a 7½ pound baby daughter born to them at seven o'clock Saturday night. Because of the raging storm it was impossible for the doctor to reach the home. . . . The snow plow could not get through the solid snow drifts . . . and the doctor attempted to walk but found it impossible because of the snow drifts. The clouds of blowing snow driven by a below zero wind made it impossible to even tell where the road was in places. The stork always seems to make his trips and is not delayed by ANY kind of weather. The worst blizzard in all history for this part of the state did not deter him this time and he arrived on schedule. Mrs. Henry Brandt, a near neighbor of the Harms, was able to get to the home and in the emergency took the place of the doctor who DIRECTED THE PROCEDURE OVER THE TELEPHONE. Everyone concerned is doing fine. Sunday morning after the storm had abated somewhat and it was possible to see, Mr. Harms drove in a bobsled and team to meet Dr. Sartor and bring him to their home. In time of need one really finds out what it means to have good neighbors and friends who will do all they can in a time of need.*

In another winter adventure, townspeople formed a "shovel brigade" to clear a path for Pierre to reach a farmhouse. A photo taken at that occasion shows more than half a dozen people trudging through deep snow, carrying shovels and supplies, to help Dr. Sartor reach the patients who needed him.

The pastor of Immanuel Lutheran Church in Titonka wrote:

> My wife and I always spoke of [Pierre] as the typical
> "Country Doctor." He was the family physician of
> the majority of my members. He was always co-oper-
> ative, always ready to help in every way possible. In
> very serious cases he would advise consulting a spe-
> cialist. It can be said of Dr. Sartor that he always took
> a personal interest in the health, welfare and life of
> his patient.

Meanwhile, Mayo Clinic remained the destination of choice:

> Little Miss Roberta Underbakke, 11, lost a part of her
> nose when a mother mare nipped her at the home of
> her parents. . . . She was taken to the Mayo clinic
> where plastic surgery restored the nose.

> Mr. Albert Meyer drove to Lakota Monday with his
> wife where they boarded the train for Rochester, Min-
> nesota. Mrs. Meyer has been a patient sufferer for
> several months and her husband has taken her to the
> Mayo hospital in search of relief. Whether she will
> submit to operations remains to be determined by the
> clinic.

> Rev. and Mrs. Killian, Mrs. H.W. Schoenlein, Rev.
> Boese of Lakota and Dr. Pierre Sartor drove to Roch-
> ester, Minn., Monday where Mrs. Killian and Mrs.
> Schoenlein will go through the Mayo clinic. The men
> returned home Monday evening. Rev. Boese went
> along to help with the driving.

After years of covering other people "going to Mayos," the editor of the *Titonka Topic* reported on his own experience:

During an Iowa blizzard, Pierre's friends formed a shovel brigade to clear a path for him to reach a patient's farmhouse.

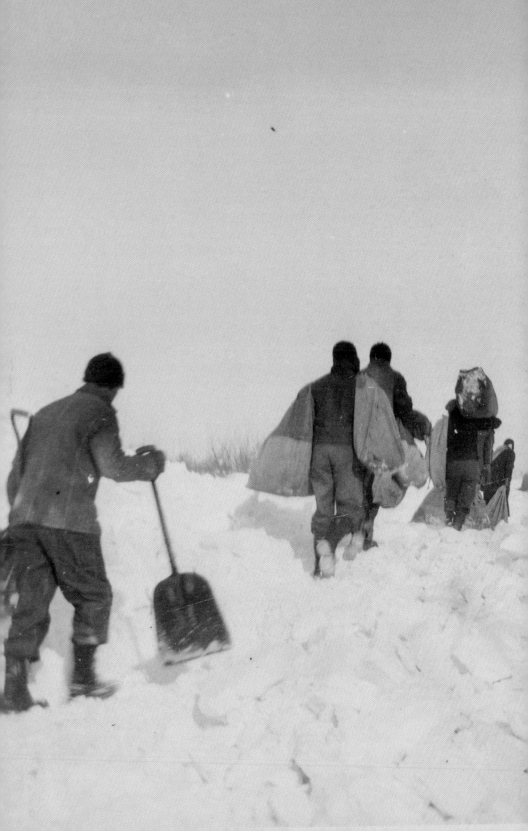

Lee O. Wolfe, editor of the Topic, spent from Thursday until Saturday night being checked up at the Mayo Clinic at Rochester, Minn. The editor was told to go home and take life easy — rest up for awhile. That is what we intend to do and will do. If you have any secrets to relate, see us at our home on Main Street where we are resting.

I should mention that in the small world of Titonka, Mr. Wolfe's wife, Inez, was the reporter who conducted the extensive interview with Pierre that I sat in on when I was 11 years old, which provided the structure of this book. Inez also was a schoolteacher — one of Guido's favorites!

These events in Pierre's practice coincided with the final years of Guido's medical training in the run-up to World War II. While conflict had begun in Asia in the early 1930s, for the Sartor family the Nazi German invasion of Poland on September 1, 1939, was especially heart-wrenching as it brought fighting to the heart of Europe.

On May 10, 1940, the Nazis invaded Luxembourg, beginning a hellish occupation that lasted more than four years. Grand Duchess Charlotte and members of the government evacuated to London to encourage resistance and demonstrate solidarity with the Allies. The Germans attempted to incorporate Luxembourg into the Nazi Reich and conscripted about 10,000 young men into the German armed forces. As part of their attempt to incorporate Luxembourg, the Nazis ordered a census that demanded information about national, ethnic and linguistic affiliation. Despite intense Nazi propaganda, the majority of respondents listed themselves as citizens of Luxembourg rather than adopt German affinity. This was a courageous affirmation of the national motto of Luxembourg, *Mir wëlle bleiwe wat mir sinn* — "We want to remain what we are."

On September 10, 1944, Luxembourg was liberated by the U.S. Army. The Nazis, however, stabilized their retreating forces along the Moselle River, which separates Luxembourg from Germany, and launched a counterattack in December. The Battle of the Bulge, as it became known, caused devastation in the north and east areas of Luxembourg. As a result of fighting and Nazi terrorism, Luxembourg suffered about 5,700 deaths in World War II, representing approximately 2% of the population. The Jewish population of Luxembourg, including refugees from other European countries, suffered extensive losses in the Holocaust.

In the fall of 1940, with the United States officially neutral but torn by the rising conflict in Europe and Asia, Guido completed his pediatrics residency. He joined the faculty and staff of Bobs Roberts Memorial Hospital, the pediatric hospital that was then affiliated with the University of Chicago.

He was delighted when Luella and Celeste, now eight years old, joined him in Chicago. The young family at last enjoyed a level of comfort: a furnished apartment, complete with maid service. In their building, above their apartment, was a penthouse where the Lawrence Welk Orchestra played each weekend. Luella and Celeste enjoyed watching the musicians come and go during the day; Luella and Guido savored their big band performances at night, under the stars.

On October 1, they moved into an apartment at 6124 South Ingleside and Celeste enrolled at the local Catholic school. This address put them near Pierre's and Mary's families in High Ridge, so they could enjoy the close bonds that stretched back several generations.

Other parallels began to form between Guido's life and Pierre's. Like his father, Guido had completed his medical training in Chicago, established a prestigious practice, and now felt the call to do something else.

Guido and Luella enjoyed Chicago, but they missed their families and the small-town, rural life. Then, in another connection to Pierre's experience, Guido learned about a job opening in Iowa. A pediatrician at Park Clinic in Mason City was entering the Army. Mason City was a thriving city, about 50 miles east of Titonka. It was an attractive opportunity. Park Clinic, like Mayo Clinic in Rochester, Minnesota, was a team-based practice of specialists. Guido would be the only pediatrician on staff. But Guido was under contract to Bobs Roberts

Hospital. And they had a lease on their apartment.

Luella took matters into her own hands. At the staff Christmas party, she approached the head of Guido's department. "I am sure I was a little naïve," she later wrote, "but I was positive that he would understand. Surely, we could sublet the apartment. It worked out that way!"

The chief agreed. Guido recognized and appreciated the opportunity, but it came at a professional cost. He later wrote: "I left the position that would mean the most to me in my entire lifetime."

On January 22, 1941, Guido, Luella and Celeste drove to their new home. Luella wrote that it was "a happy happy day" and underlined "happy" twice. It was 22 degrees below zero and the highways were coated with ice. They drove to the Iowa prairie, recreating his parents' journey to what Pierre had considered the Wild West.

Change was all around. As Guido and his family settled in Mason City, the United States became increasingly drawn into the conflicts in Europe and Asia. Less than a year after Guido established his practice in Mason City, the Japanese attacked Pearl Harbor on December 7, 1941, and the United States entered World War II.

On April 24, 1942, I was born, the second child of Guido and Luella. My name is Mary Elizabeth, in honor of Mamie Murphy; I was born three days after her birthday. My parents sent photos to Mamie, who replied with enthusiasm, continuing her longtime correspondence with the family. Pierre noted that Mary was also Grandma Sartor's name, and so a good choice all around. In the years to come, Guido and Luella were blessed with additional children: Julie Anne, born January 28, 1949; and Robert Pierre, born December 19, 1952.

A few months after I was born, my father drove to Ohio for the funeral of my namesake, Mamie Murphy. Guido walked down the church aisle with Frank Murphy, much like a son.

Guido's own father, Pierre, continued his medical practice in Titonka. As in World War I, many doctors were called to military duty, so his services were in great demand. During the war years, Pierre was past the age of retirement and considered elderly, but still going strong. According to a newspaper report from the year he turned 70, "Dr. Pierre Sartor fell on the ice and cracked some ribs," but this was only a temporary setback. A member of the community at that time wrote: "I vividly recall how he stayed at the bedside of a member of my family through an entire night, despite his advancing age."

Guido, for his part, established himself as "an excellent pediatrician," in the words of Dr. Art McMahon, a colleague at the Park Clinic. Dr. Richard Munns, who practiced in Hampton, Iowa, said he referred patients to Guido "with 100 percent good results." Pierre's influence shows in Dr. McMahon's description of Guido: "a gentleman from the old school — very professional, quiet and unassuming." Dr. Van Hunt, also a colleague of Guido's at Park Clinic, said Guido "was esteemed" by the community. "He loved his family, his church. He was an honorable man." In a newspaper interview, Dr. Hunt also recounted other qualities that people who knew Swifty Sartor would recognize:

> On a humorous note, Hunt said he was aware of one weakness Sartor had: Cadillacs.
>
> "He always drove Cadillacs," Hunt said with a chuckle. "I can remember about how he wanted to take the car out and 'see what it could do.'
>
> "He found a short stretch of road near Titonka that did not have any intersecting roads, so he could take it out safely."
>
> Still, a neighbor complained about someone driving 90 mph down the rural road.

Sartors, Titonka,

VOWS OF 1898 RENEWED IN CHURCH RITES

By Inez Wolfe.

Dr. and Mrs. Pierre Sartor, Titonka, celebrated their golden wedding anniversary this week. The picture shown here was taken at their home Sunday after they returned from Algona, where a family dinner was served at the Algona hotel.

Doctor and Mrs. Sartor were married Oct. 20, 1898, at Chicago on the bride's 19th birthday anniversary. The ceremony was performed by the Rev. Father Reutershof, at St. Henry's parish.

Mrs. Sartor came to Bancroft in December 1901, when Mary, the eldest child, was a baby. Doctor Sartor had come in November, but in February 1918 moved to Titonka where there is 17 years, since resided. They lived there 17

Six Sartor Children.

The couple had six children, but Anthony, beloved youngest ("Tinny"), died at 14 from a heart condition.

The other children were all at the anniversary party: Mary (Mrs. Oesterreicher, a teacher at Titonka); Magdalene (Mrs. J. E. Bleich), Britt, a former primary teacher; Dr. Guido, pediatrician on the Park hospital staff, Mason City; Mercedes (Mrs. Joseph Coyle), Chicago, a registered nurse; and Alice (Mrs. Mason at Charles City. There are six grandchildren.

All of the Sartor children and the families were present Sunday morning at early mass at St. Joseph's church, Wesley, when the parents renewed their marriage vows.

Dr. and Mrs. Pierre Sartor

Photo by Missal

TITONKIANS, BANCROFTERS, and a wide circle of other friends will have no difficulty in recognizing this picture of the veteran physician and his wife, who are celebrating their fifty years of wedded loyalty and happiness ding. Most of their fifty years of wedded loyalty and happiness ha been spent in Kossuth county, and as old age impends both are st in good health and much more active than many other couples their time.

A Song for Pierre

Titonka, Iowa
1946-1958

IN MANY RESPECTS, THE POST-WORLD WAR II YEARS
were especially satisfying for Pierre and Mary.

An article about Pierre in the *Journal of Iowa State Medical So-ciety* reported: "Dr. Sartor says he still has 'a pretty busy prac-tice,' part in Titonka and part in the surrounding rural area and
at Bancroft."

This was quite an understatement, judging by comments
from patients and friends who described Pierre in his 70s:

> *Our offices are but four doors apart, I see him practi-
> cally every day, and greatly enjoy his friendship. . . .
> He is active and alert, like a man of 30 years his ju-
> nior. . . . Only a couple of years ago, he was president
> of our Chamber of Commerce, and during his year in
> that office we had one of the most active years in the
> Chamber[']s existence.*

―――――――

*Dr. Pierre and Mary Sartor celebrated their golden wedding anniver-
sary in 1948.*

After all these years of doctoring and community ser-
vice, his step today is as light and his answer to calls
day or night is as prompt as ever, making it hard to
believe he has served more than half a century. We
deem it a great privilege to know him as a doctor, a
counselor and a friend.

Their wedding anniversary celebrations were publicized year after year in the *Titonka Topic* with special attention to their golden anniversary in 1948. At their renewal of vows, Mary carried her First Communion prayer book — the same book she had carried on her wedding day and which other brides in our family have carried across the ensuing decades.

The celebration dinner was spirited. The Chicago relatives had sent their regrets — then, in a delightful surprise to Pierre and Mary, they attended en masse. A reel-to-reel tape recording was made of the event. Voices are mixed amid the sounds of people laughing and talking, the rattle of dishes, songs from the Spanish-American War era of Pierre and Mary's wedding and what seems to be great delight in the fine wines of Luxembourg. Pierre can be heard describing his Atlantic Ocean journey on the tramp steamer and Mary mentions one of her bridesmaids. Pierre's phrase "keep agoing" is audible and Alice calls her mother, Mary, "the most dignified of the crew."

The community shared a deep appreciation of Pierre. There was also the awareness — due to his advancing age and the evolution of medicine toward specialization as represented in Guido's career — that Pierre's model of care, the general practitioner country doctor, was beloved but increasingly historic.

Pierre became a fixture at parades. For several years, he rode in a horse-drawn buggy, the classic picture of a small-town physician. Pierre pulled his Prince Albert coat out of storage for these occasions. It was still a symbol of his status, but at this point Pierre was most proud of the fact that it remained in excellent condition and still fit him perfectly.

Along with his decades-long delight in that coat, Pierre's quirks and charm were a legend in the community, as well as in the family. He accepted many honors in those years, including "Dr. Sartor Day," a celebration attended by hundreds of patients and friends from Titonka and the surrounding area. The sponsoring committee represented a half-dozen organizations in which Pierre and Mary were active. At the end of the festivities, Pierre serenaded the bevy of guests with his trademark song, "Home on the Range."

No matter how often the invitations came, each card, every letter, all the phone calls caught him by surprise. Guido cherished the twinkle in his father's eye, the way Pierre blended several languages when he got excited, and the warmth Pierre felt when the community expressed its love for him.

These honors came in response to the dedication Pierre had shown to his patients over many years. His dedication was so strong, in fact, that Pierre nearly missed two of the most important milestones of his career.

On September 16, 1946, the Kossuth County Medical Society planned a gala event to recognize Pierre's 50-year career as a doctor. The Iowa Medical Society sent a plaque. The Winandys sent flowers. It was to be at Schutter's Café in Titonka. As Pierre was getting ready to leave home for the event, a man burst in the Sartors' front door. He had a severe nosebleed.

Pierre knew what he had to do. With a quick grasp of Mary's hand and a worried goodbye, Pierre led the man to his car for the 15-mile drive to Algona. The specialized equipment he needed was at the hospital there.

The hours passed quickly. Pierre had the man admitted to the hospital and became absorbed in caring for him. I don't know what he did to stop the man's nosebleed or why it took so long. It's likely that after the crisis passed, Pierre stayed with the patient to keep him comfortable: the same labor-intensive, holistic care Pierre had performed during the influenza pandemic and many times since then.

By the time Pierre got around to checking his watch, the time of the gala event had arrived and gone. The guest of honor was a no-show.

It was past midnight when Pierre arrived home. As he turned the car onto his street, he slowed down, puzzled. Cars filled his driveway and were parked up and down the street. He had to park some distance away and walk to his house. At this late hour, the windows were aglow.

Mary opened the back door. She was hosting a party, she said, and ushered him into the house, which was crowded with his friends and colleagues. Earlier in the evening, when it became clear that Pierre was not coming to the café, the event planners called Mary; she explained he was tending to an emergency. So the party came to him, awaiting his arrival. For the plaque presentation, a newspaper photographer took a picture of the doctors gathered in Pierre and Mary's dining room. Amid the congratulations and good cheer, flashbulbs popped and sizzled to the floor.

As the *Titonka Topic* explained:

> *When the hour had arrived for the doctor's party, the guest of honor was missing. An investigation proved the doctor had gone to an Algona hospital with a patient and he did not return until the dinner was over and the guests had repaired to the Sartor home. Next morning Dr. Sartor said that was only an ordinary happening in the life of the country doctor.*

Pierre used his oft-spoken words: *I was needed.*

But Pierre was no ordinary country doctor, a fact that was underscored six years later in remarkably similar circumstances.

Pierre had been a loyal member of the Kossuth County Medical Society for decades, and duly noted its monthly meeting for March 1952 on his calendar. Guido came from Mason City to Titonka to attend the meeting that evening as well, for reasons he did not make quite clear, but Pierre didn't press the matter. As a respected pediatrician, Guido was always welcomed by his peers and colleagues.

Then it happened again — a patient in crisis — Pierre's plans upended. This time, the patient had an excruciating earache, which must have triggered special empathy from Pierre, given his childhood experience, and of course a call to action.

Again . . . the trip to the hospital, the hours spent at the patient's bedside, the long, late return home. Pierre regretted missing the meeting, but he must have consoled himself that it wasn't the first time he had to cancel on late notice and, at least on this night, he wasn't the guest of honor.

Again . . . his surprise must have been profound when he turned onto his street to see cars parked all around and his house blazing with light.

Again . . . Mary met him at the door, ever the accomplished hostess. This time, however, she was mum about what was going on as she led him into the crowd of physicians.

Dr. C.R. Cretzmeyer, Pierre's friend since he first visited Bancroft shortly after graduating from medical school, commanded everyone's attention. As the room fell silent, he announced: *Tonight the physicians of the Kossuth County Medical Society have nominated Dr. Pierre Sartor to be Iowa Medical Society's General Practitioner of the Year.*

The nomination was entirely appropriate. Pierre at this point was the oldest practicing physician in Kossuth County and often referred to as the "dean" of doctors in the area. Nevertheless, Pierre was astonished at the news. "Astonished" is the word that Guido used for his father's reaction. Pierre's face was frozen. He could not step through his dining room door. If Pierre used one of his signature oaths — *By golly!* — one can understand his surprise.

The doctors explained the nomination process. Each member of the Kossuth County Medical Society was to write a letter of recommendation, stating why Dr. Pierre Sartor should be selected above all the doctors who would be nominated from across the state. Pierre's patients, neighbors and friends in the community would also write letters on his behalf.

As dozens of endorsement letters arrived over the next few days and weeks, Pierre's eldest child, May, collected them into a book that the Kossuth County Medical Society submitted to the Iowa Medical Society in Des Moines. Even today, with the passage of many years, the words speak volumes about the respect that many people held for Pierre: "It was not done for the love of money nor worldly goods and achievement but simply for the love of mankind and his desire to fulfill his mission in life as God gave him the talent and time to do so."

Dr. George F. Dolmage, Pierre's colleague during the influenza pandemic and throughout the years that followed, sent a handwritten letter to Guido: "Mrs. Dolmage has often made the remark that 'Dr. Sartor may not have a lot of money, but I know he has lots of good friends.'"

The *Titonka Topic* had some fun along the same lines with a tongue-in-cheek article about unreasonable complaints: "You can complain because Doc Sartor doesn't drive nights when he did that night driving many[,] many years bringing babies into the world that are not yet paid for."

Warm, humorous and sincere, the outpouring of comments can be summarized in these words: "I am sure that a great many people can say that their life was made a little easier and that this world was just a little better place in which to live because Dr. Pierre Sartor has lived here."

The Iowa Medical Society received nominations from throughout the state. The recipient of this honor would be announced at the society's meeting at the Fort Des Moines Hotel in the state capital. Pierre and Guido attended and never forgot the surprise and delight when Dr. Pierre Sartor was named the Iowa General Practitioner of the Year on April 29, 1953.

It was the crowning achievement of Pierre's career, but my sister Celeste recalls that after expressing his heartfelt and humble appreciation, Pierre said he had to leave after lunch. He had to get back to his patients.

Along with "Doctor of the Year," Pierre sometimes was described as "Iowa's Country Doctor." The *Iowa Medical Journal* and newspapers throughout the Midwest carried stories about his life.

Guido put copies of the letters and newspaper clippings into a portfolio for safekeeping. Guido was pleased and honored to

As the classic "country doctor," Pierre became a fixture at parades. He enjoyed wearing the elegant frock coat he had purchased decades before.

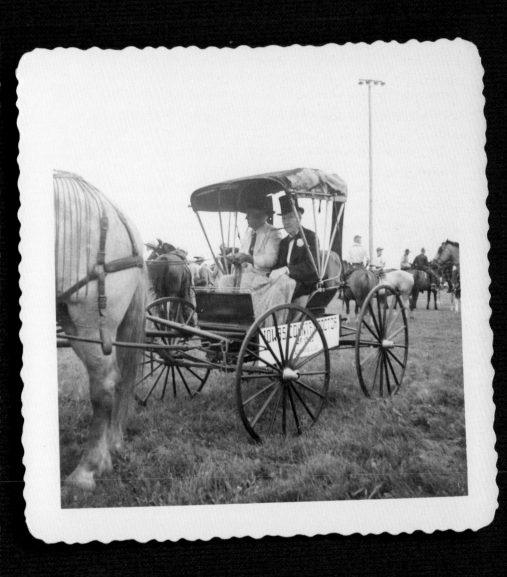

receive many letters from his own medical colleagues and friends, from physicians and patients throughout northern Iowa and from fellow members of the Iowa Pediatric Society, congratulating him on his father's honor.

Through testimonials, coverage in the news media and events at which he was honored, Pierre's life story was becoming widely known. It also was around this time that Pierre wrote his memoir, "Thrills of my life — specifically my 'Flu Life.'"

The handwritten manuscript that survives is not dated and it's not clear if Pierre had other versions of its content. "Thrills of my life" seems to have been written as a speech and we know that Pierre addressed audiences on multiple occasions after he was nominated and received the award.

After one event, the *Algona Advance* made a lighthearted observation: "It was a perfect day for the doctor . . . he wasn't called away to care for a patient!"

On several occasions, Dr. Cretzmeyer introduced Pierre when he delivered the "Thrills of my life" speech. Dr. Cretzmeyer knew how to engage his audience. He described Pierre as "the little roly-poly cherub we are gathered here to honor today" and commended Pierre with the words of Robert Louis Stevenson: "'There are men and classes of men that rise above the common herd. The physician invariably belongs to this group.' . . . May you live many years to continue your errands of mercy."

New Horizons magazine featured Pierre on its cover. Published by the Iowa division of the American Cancer Society, it was distributed to 215,000 families throughout the state: "The experiences that Dr. Sartor recalls most vividly — and the ones in which he takes the greatest pride — occurred during the nationwide influenza epidemic of 1918 and 1919." The journal also cited the data that Pierre presented in his memoir: "More than a thousand of his patients were stricken with the disease at one time or another during the winter. . . . Though influenza was more frequently fatal then than it ever has been since, Dr. Sartor lost only five patients."

The widespread coverage of Pierre's story seems to have kindled particular memories for one of his patients. The last case study in his memoir is about how "Tony's wife" cared for an ill woman whose daughter, "about four years old," was also ill. Pierre wrote:

> Mother looked at me and said, pointing to the little girl, 'Doctor, if you make that one well again, you can ask of me anything you wish for.' 'All right,' I said. 'I want you and your daughter some day to sing for me.'

We don't know exactly what happened or when, but sometime before Pierre wrote his memoir, while his name was prominent in state and local news, he must have been contacted by his former patient. The denouement of his speech would have been intriguing to any audience: "The mother was a good singer, and the little girl, grown up and by now a wonderful singer, can have a chance to do what mother promised at my next 82nd birthday, if the good Lord so will it."

Pierre entitled his memoir "Thrills of my life — specifically my 'Flu Life.'" What he hinted at in the memoir led directly to the *surprise* of his life.

Pierre's 82nd birthday was Sunday, August 23, 1953. That year also marked the 60th anniversary of his arrival in the United States. We celebrated his birthday the day before, Saturday the 22nd.

I remember the day. It was brutally hot, as an Iowa summer can be. The sun burned through air as thick as pudding.

My father honked the horn of our car as we arrived. He and my mother brought a cake, the kind of confection you get from a bakery for special occasions, with Pierre's name in sugary script. My sister Celeste had returned to Iowa State College in Ames, Iowa, to start her senior year. That made me, at age 11, the oldest child in our family that day. I rushed to Grandpa for a hug. Pierre was wearing a necktie and a white shirt tucked into his trademark high-waisted trousers, which were held up by suspenders. Then I snuggled next to Grandma on the davenport; the hem of Mary's voile dress fluttered in the warm air that circulated from a nearby fan.

Pierre next hugged Julie, age 4½. Settling into his chair, he swung Julie up to his lap. This told us it was her turn for Pierre's familiar ritual with his grandchildren and other favored youngsters. It began with Pierre and the child on his lap fixing their gaze one to another.

The rest of our group fell silent as Pierre commenced a mysterious incantation. He spoke in the dialect from the old country, maybe half a dozen lines in a soothing rhythm, his fingertip stroking her palm with each phrase. He built excitement by his tone and with his eyes. Even though no grandchild understood the language of Luxembourg, we were enthralled.

Then came the crescendo, as Pierre's voice soared into a high trill that sounded like *Deedle-deedle-deedle-dention*! Julie squealed, as every child did during Pierre's performance, because at that moment, a sparkling silver half dollar dropped into her palm, from — where?

Pierre's magic was on display. It was a rare gift, far more valuable than the coins he distributed.

My brother, Bobby — Robert Pierre — was next. At seven months of age, he had been all a-wiggle while Julie had her turn and nudged in as close as he could. A few moments later and he, too, was clutching a coin from Grandpa.

After Pierre's magic performance, we youngsters headed out for the porch. Guido headed for the kitchen, following a tradition of his own. He clinked open the tin doors of the cupboard and soon returned carrying glasses filled with suds. Pierre balanced his stein. How the beer sloshed with the adults' chatter, and then Pierre's glass sloshed over. *Good beer doesn't stain*, Guido said, and they all laughed. As if Pierre and the ladies hadn't heard that one before.

The talk turned to crops . . . hog futures . . . who might stop by later for refreshments. As their conversation subsided, the radio, playing in the background, took over. Given the headlines of that time, the announcer may have described the polio epidemic then underway; the Salk vaccine was still in the future.

Whereas the influenza Pierre had fought occurred in fall and winter, polio struck in warm weather. "Polio summer" was the dreaded time when movie theaters, beaches and amusement parks were closed by official order to limit the disease from spreading — another example of the isolation philosophy Pierre had called for decades earlier. Just as Pierre, a country doctor, was on the front lines when influenza struck his rural patients, Guido, a pediatrician, was in the thick of fighting polio, the scourge of children. To receive specialty training, Guido enrolled in a class at the Sister Kenny Institute, sponsored by the University of Minnesota.

But this was Pierre's birthday, and the conversation found its way back to cake and celebration. The front screen door banged open, and the postman entered, closing the door behind him to keep out the heat. He was a friend of the family and in Titonka that level of familiarity was understood and accepted, particularly on an occasion like Pierre's birthday. The postman and Pierre had a jolly exchange during the handover of a large assortment of cards and letters.

Pierre leaned on the wall while he rifled through the stack of mail. Then one card brought him to a halt. His eyes watered. Pierre went to the dining room and placed the cards on his desk. He pulled his lockbox down from the shelf, not in a hurry, even though everyone had stopped talking. I remember him saying "anno domini" — Latin for "in the year of the Lord."

Guido, looky here, he said, loudly. And he did mean to startle. He laid one card on the desk and flattened it open so Guido could see. *It is from the baby in the mother's bed, now grown*, he said.

I don't recall what was on the card and it has not survived among our family artifacts. But it had a connection to the memoir Pierre had recently written: "The little girl, grown up and by now a wonderful singer, can have a chance to do what mother promised at my next 82nd birthday, if the good Lord so will it."

The card announced that the woman Pierre had met as a sick toddler would come to his home that very day to sing for him and settle her mother's long-ago debt.

Pierre ended his memoir with the story of the sick toddler, now an accomplished musician, who had "a chance to do what mother promised" by singing at his birthday.

The final written words in the narrative are "if the good Lord so will it," and I believe it is most fitting that the good Lord, as in so many aspects of Pierre's life, did indeed "will it," allowing patient and physician to reconnect decades after they first met in a cold farmhouse.

For Pierre Sartor, such a gift of music and gratitude was the most meaningful payment of all.

Pierre was delighted at the progress of Guido's career, which represented the increased specialization of medicine.

Dr. Sartor President of Iowa Pediatric Society

Dr. G. J. Sartor of Mason City has been installed as president of the Iowa Pediatric Society of the Iowa State Medical Society. Previously president-elect of the pediatricians, he has served for five years on the executive committee of the Iowa Pediatric Society.

Dr. Sartor also has been appointed chairman of the pediatric section of the Iowa State Medical Society for 1959 by Dr. Walter Ahrens, president of the state society. In he be responsible for the medical programs presented at the general session of the Iowa State Medical Society and of the Iowa Pediatric

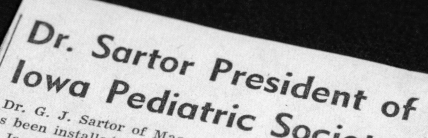

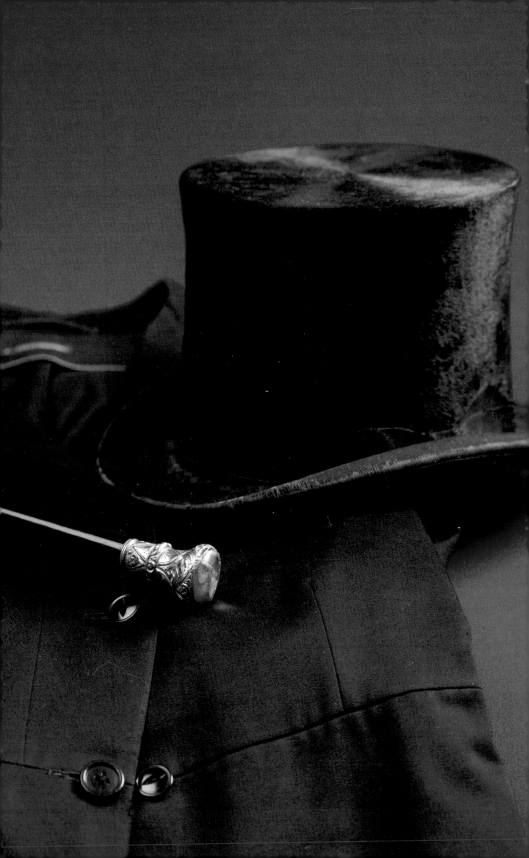

The Lockbox — A Continuing Journey

AND WHAT WAS IN THE LOCKBOX when I opened it decades after that memorable birthday party?

Not the pebbles, bird wings and clouds that I imagined when I peeked into it at age four. Instead, I saw items from Pierre, my grandfather, and Guido, my father, that connected to the stories I'd heard over many years, and which brought those memories to life.

There was a business card with a picture of a big baby in honor of the 19-pound infant Pierre delivered in Chicago.

A letter from Luxembourg.

Three pages tied in string: Pierre's birth certificate, which he translated into German, French and English.

The letters that Pierre's brother Ferdinand wrote in 1893, inviting him to America.

Pierre's medical school diploma, still wrapped in its delivery package. Pierre was proud of his professional calling, but he never had the diploma framed for display.

Pierre's top hat and gold-headed walking stick, inscribed to recognize him as General Practitioner of the Year, symbolize his commitment to excellence.

The record of patients Pierre saw during the three years he practiced in Chicago, 1896 to 1899. Those who paid and who did not, the services he provided, what he charged. Baby deliveries were $3; consulting appointments were $1.

A list of Pierre and Mary's grandchildren, with their baptismal dates, signed and dated 1941; Pierre was 70 at the time. Guido described seeing him write the list from memory, even the middle names — even the godparents' names.

Pierre's memoir: "Thrills of my life."

An article by Charles Mayo, M.D., in a medical journal. Pierre's handwritten addition, "The Mayo Miracle," showing his high regard for Mayo Clinic.

As for Guido?

There were humorous sketches that he drew of his college classmates in the 1920s, letters from Mamie Murphy, his records from treating children in the polio epidemic and a poignant document entitled "My greatest disappointment" — his account of a girl whose condition he could not treat, despite seeking help from other specialists. Reading it, I realized I had met this girl when I was 11 or 12 years old — the only patient my father ever brought to our home. She was my age and I wanted to play with her, but she was too frail. Daddy treated her with great kindness and made her feel like an honored guest. She died soon after, and my father always cherished a gift she gave him — a hand-painted statue of the Madonna.

There was also a small book. It symbolizes the enduring bond between Guido and Pierre.

They had a remarkable relationship, characterized by mutual respect as well as love. Pierre had a high regard for his own father, Mathias, who sacrificed and planned carefully for him. But Pierre's contact with Mathias was limited — barely past childhood, Pierre left home for a year of medical treatment, followed by nearly a decade of boarding school education and then emigration from the homeland, never to return.

Pierre had two sons of his own and one of them, Anthony, died as an adolescent.

It was with Guido, then, that Pierre established a close father-son relationship. He had a similar bond with his daughters.

On their trips together during the influenza pandemic, Pierre mentored and taught Guido, but in the years that followed, Pierre looked up to his physician son. My sister Celeste describes how Pierre admired Guido as representing the new generation of specialized medical professionals. At Pierre's urging, Guido frequently quizzed Pierre on medical topics — Pierre wanted to be sure he was up to date with the current state of knowledge. As Celeste will tell you, Grandpa passed each test with flying colors.

Guido, for his part, expressed solidarity with his father in a way that Pierre always treasured. As a Christmas present in 1938, he gave Pierre the book *Don't Believe It! Says the Doctor* by August Thomen, M.D.; according to its subtitle, the book dispelled *False Notions, Errors, Misperceptions and Misinformation pertaining to Health and Hygiene* — the commitment to excellence that Pierre brought to the care of his patients, which Guido continued in his own career.

In presenting this gift, Guido signed it "G.J. Sartor, M.D," adding his affiliation with the Department of Pediatrics, University of Chicago Clinics. It was a gift from one medical colleague to another, as well as from son to father. The love and respect it conveyed symbolized the bond between them. Pierre kept the book in the lockbox and, after Pierre died, Guido did also, and that lockbox eventually passed to me. Both men knew the inscription by heart:

> *To Father,*
> *Whose vast experience I wish were inheritable; if so,*
> *I would ask of him no more.*

Dr. Pierre Sartor died August 5, 1958, shortly before his 87th birthday. Toward the end of his life, he and Mary were both patients at Park Hospital in Mason City. After his passing, Mary told a friend who visited her in the hospital that she wondered, *How long until the Lord will call?* That call came on November 1, 1958, shortly after her 79th birthday and their 60th wedding anniversary. For years thereafter, a room in Park Hospital was named in their honor.

My parents had their own experience of caregiving for each other, setting an example of devotion that lives on for us. In the late summer of 1989, my mother, Luella, 80 years old, went next door to care for a dog whose owners were away. As she was leaving, she fell about 10 steps off their back deck. She broke her right wrist and left ankle. Guido, my father, was not home at the time. Mom had to crawl across the neighbor's yard and get herself into the side door of our house until Guido came home. She never walked on her own again and was confined to their home for the rest of her life.

In his mid-80s, Daddy cared for her for the next six years until she died on February 22, 1995. Too often in those years, someone would tell Guido that they felt sorry for him — he shouldn't be taking on that responsibility. One day, *he* had too much. My father got as angry as anyone had ever seen him. It was painful to watch him back up to the fireplace for support, and he spoke loud and clear, his voice trembling with emotion:

> *Every morning I wake up and come straight down-*
> *stairs to find her. I sit in my chair across from her and*
> *I thank God that we have another day together.*

Dr. Guido Sartor lived exactly nine years after his beloved Luella died. He passed quietly in his sleep the night of February 22-23, 2004. I don't know for a fact if my father realized the date, but in my heart I'm sure he did.

In the development of this book, my friends at Mayo Clinic introduced me to the phrase "miracle of relationships," which Sister Ellen Whelan coined when she wrote a history of the Franciscan Sisters at Saint Marys Hospital and their long association with Mayo. That phrase is equally true of Pierre and Guido Sartor, and their connections to family, patients, colleagues and community.

I thank you for sharing this time with my family, and I wonder what "miracle of relationships" you have in your life. I wish you all the best as you follow dreams of your own and fill the lockbox of your memories with stories that are meaningful to you and yours.

About the Author

Mary Beth Sartor Obermeyer brings a lifetime of experience to the writing of this book.

As the granddaughter of Dr. Pierre Sartor and the daughter of Dr. Guido Sartor, Beth grew up listening to family stories, particularly about the 1918 influenza pandemic. She paid such careful attention that her mother, Luella, declared Beth was "taking inventory." These stories, augmented by extensive research, are the foundation of *When Winter Came*.

Beth graduated from Iowa State University in 1964 with a degree in journalism. In 1965, she married Twin Cities architect Dr. Thomas Obermeyer and they became the parents of Mark and Kristin.

Beth's career connects her achievements as a performing artist, entrepreneur and journalist. Among many honors, she returned to Iowa State University as a Professional in Residence and served as a keynote speaker at Iowa State University, the University of Minnesota and Drake University.

Beth spent her youth in Mason City, Iowa, the setting of Meredith Willson's *The Music Man*, and flourished as a dancer at local and regional events. Her memoir of those experiences, *The Days of Song and Lilacs*, was a finalist for the Midwest Book Awards.

While on the faculty of the Minnesota Dance Theatre, Beth

soloed with the Minnesota Orchestra. She also performed solo with celebrities Christopher Plummer and Garrison Keillor, as well as with Gregory Hines to promote his film *Tap*.

The founder of TA DA! Special Events, Beth produced and publicized public extravaganzas. They included an ensemble of 1,801 tap dancers who performed on Hennepin Avenue in Minneapolis to open an arts center and the World's Largest Marching Band — 2,512 musicians strong — guest-conducted by Meredith Willson. Five of Beth's events earned Guinness World Records. Beth and her events received four CUE Awards from the Minneapolis Committee for the Urban Environment, and one of her events earned the Business in the Arts Award from *Forbes* magazine. Beth's books *The Biggest Dance: A Miracle on Concrete* and *Big! World Records in the Street* describe the unique power of the arts to bring people together.

In 1988, Beth produced her last large-scale public event, the Minnesota Festival of the Book, a weeklong, statewide celebration of literature for readers of all ages and backgrounds. This fueled her interest in writing and took Beth back to the stories of her youth — leading to the day when she found her grandfather's handwritten memoir of a long-ago pandemic and discovered how he brought help and hope to the people who needed him most.

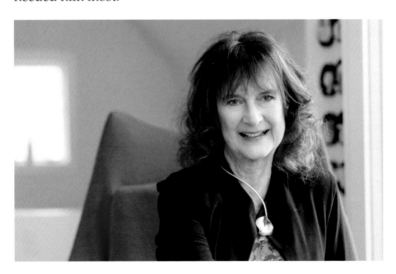

Acknowledgments

Mary Beth Sartor Obermeyer, author

I must begin by reflecting on the many contributions of my husband, Tom Obermeyer, to the publication of this book. An author himself, Tom understood the space that a manuscript holds in a storytelling brain. The characters in my story never went to sleep — they didn't know night from day. The scenes were vivid to me, and never shut down. Even when my pencil became a nub, when Tom and I escaped for a walk, the characters would whisper to me. My ear would grow hot, and off on a sidetrack I would go. A partner with that kind of patience is a gift!

As an architect, Tom also predicted that I would eat space. Without notice, I would own the living room, surrounded by a tornado of papers. He stood by while the ball chair by the fireplace, filled with notebooks and files and where I could evaporate for hours, became my refuge. He even tolerated spare bookshelves on rollers stashed by windows and blocking doors to the balcony or deck. This definitely was not in his blueprint.

And then, when a manuscript finally emerged and all that research could be contained in his hand, or mine — I was gone! Tom drove me to bookstores and venues to talk to readers about my story. He read six subsequent drafts. Most importantly, he helped me wind down at the end of each day with a meal at a restaurant, a picnic, a bike ride through the park or a leisurely walk.

Unlike my book characters, Tom did not change. He was steady to the end.

I am also grateful to a larger world of family, friends and historians, people who stepped in on the journey of this amazing tale. And yet, before I bring each to mind, I stand for a moment to acknowledge — in awe — how fortunate we are that the story passed through us, one generation to the next and to the next. How very close the narrative came to disappearing in time.

My grandfather lived to be almost 90. I was 17 when he died, just old enough to realize and appreciate his spirit. My father, who also would become a doctor, lived to almost 100. By then, I was showing him early stand-alone scenes for the book. And when I was a mere 80 years old, I received an opportunity to collaborate with Mayo Clinic Press to bring my grandfather's story to print. I believe something greater than all of us was at play. We barely overlapped, each stepping in our own time, not knowing what we carried.

At the same time, I fully understand that nothing could be told had my grandfather, Dr. Pierre Sartor, not written his memoir of the flu pandemic of 1918 and kept his folded notes in the lockbox with other important papers of his life. For all of that I am so very grateful.

This telling of my grandfather's story might not have happened had the Friends of the St. Paul Public Library not hired me to direct the first Minnesota Festival of the Book in 1988. It changed my life's direction. I was inspired, but I didn't know what I wanted to write! I thank Scott Walker, publisher at Graywolf Press, who gave me Brenda Ueland's book *If You Want to Write*, along with some advice: "Just write, same time, every day."

But I needed more. To the Loft Literary Center I went, to learn to tell a story. There I met Kate St. Vincent Vogl. She stayed with my story about my grandfather and would edit the sixth draft for pace. She still encourages me every step of the journey. My story would not have left home without her.

I also started a year of Saturday morning creative writing classes at St. Catherine University in St. Paul, and Jack Galloway was my instructor. His first praise came months in, for what would two decades later become the opening of my third book.

It was a favorite instructor from my alma mater Iowa State University, Professor James Schwartz, who suggested — seemingly out of nowhere — "I think your best story will be about your grandfather and your father."

In 1995, five months after our 27-year-old son, Mark, died in a tragic accident and a month after my mother died, I backed up in time. I visited my father often, each time bringing written excerpts about my grandfather. My father would greet me at the door, only to look to my hands, to see if I had new pages. He would disappear into his den to read while Tom and I waited. When he emerged, he'd nod, give me a book or two and send me off to explore new directions. It reminded me of eighth grade when he took me to the library and showed me how to research a paper. Or when my mother sat me on the davenport in the den at age four and had me read aloud every night.

An enormous resource for me at this time were the reel-to-reel tapes my dad made of my grandfather telling stories. They were replayed frequently throughout my childhood.

Unfortunately, I don't have many of them today, but the stories stayed with me, and I often went to sleep at night to the lull and laughter of Grandpa Sartor. In the years until he reached almost 100, my father never stopped telling me stories about his life and my grandfather's life, just as he had since I was young.

As my journey continued, I ended up in a writing group that was special, the Caribou Scribblers, with classmates from a Loft class. How we wrote and pondered away over our writings. And we vowed that we wouldn't stop until each finished a book.

The next push came when my husband died unexpectedly. Weeks later Kate St. Vincent Vogl suggested an author group to provide some distraction. We met in the home of Jane Resh Thomas, a well-known and experienced writer, editor and teacher. For the next year, every other Monday morning, we read our chapters and received feedback. Jane could dissect pages just by listening; she needed no hard copy. Without Jane, I might have veered off track; my life had changed in large ways. Also in the group were Shari Albers and Julie Evans. We still track each other and cheer each manuscript submission. And we analyze any response, especially criticism! Jane gave us all a morning to drop out of the world and watch the stars.

Back home, I dived into research, gaining a new appreciation of its importance. In 2019, 40 years after my first trip to my grandfather's beloved Luxembourg, I returned to learn more. Again, the Luxie hospitality glowed. We visited Pierre's birthplace in the tiny village of Berbourg. The sweet and passionate stories my grandfather had told me, often recorded by my father on reel-to-reel tape, came full circle. Luxembourg was as beautiful and the people as caring as he'd described. Special thanks to relatives Emile Weydert and Andree Hoffeld-Rischette and to Monternach Mayor Jean-Pierre Hoffmann and retired Assistant Mayor Albert Schumacher. On that trip, I became a Luxie citizen, along with my daughter, Kristin, and grandsons, Jack and Brooks. During our travels, we also visited the Van Gogh Museum in Amsterdam and viewed drawings set at the time of Pierre's childhood in nearby Belgium, a visual grounding for my story.

Home again in Minneapolis, I became friends with second and third cousins in my grandmother's Winandy family, Jean Evinger and Marlene Harrolle. We exchanged photos of the immigrant family of our shared beginnings. They were familiar with the Winandy homes and adept at ancestral research. We bonded, recognizing a common energy — and were persistent.

Family members and friends were integral to writing this story. They sent newspaper articles, family photos and family memories of generations past. My sister Julie and her husband, David, transferred files onto CDs. My brother Robert, who has great research skills, performed background research and verified details. My older sister, Celeste, shared some of my grandfather's memorabilia, including his Prince Albert coat, his prayer book and a medical text. My nephew Bob Roth spent countless hours gathering family history. William Schaeffer, great-grandson of Ferdinand Sartor, sent photos and stories of Ferdinand and Margaretha's family. And William's daughter, Karen Monson, wrote of Chicago days with her Sartor grandmother.

From college friends, I received handwritten accounts of the 1918 flu and World War I, written by their ancestors. Both events gave me insight into the times of my book.

My daughter, Kristin Quinby, was my first reader, through many drafts, an astute eye for character development. She's also a brilliant little techie, who knows how to keep my computer running. My niece Jean Roth Marinelli read over countless scenes for me; invaluable in her way with words. Dr. Ronald C. Hansen, who as a child was a patient of my father's and became inspired to become a physician, read the text and offered valuable insights.

Even my neighbors would give me the opportunity to share my story. By their eyes I sensed the peaks and valleys in my narrative. Once, Cathy Polasky burst through my door to package and rush to the post office a timeline for the book that had somehow gotten away from me. It covered my entire dining room table! In addition, I was trying to draw maps, of Luxembourg and Iowa and the Chicago area, which is not my forte. "I'm going to call you the Rand McNally of Mayo Clinic Publishing," my editor lightheartedly responded.

The most pivotal event in my journey came when David Unowsky, owner of the former Hungry Mind Bookstore in St. Paul, saw posts on my Facebook page about my manuscript, by then in its seventh draft. He connected me to Mayo Clinic Press and my amazing editor Matthew Dacy.

In the midst of the COVID-19 pandemic, I met with eight

members of Mayo Clinic in a Zoom meeting, and these individuals would become the team that launched *When Winter Came*. A new mission was born at that meeting: "Collaborate!" Soon we would stand shoulder to shoulder, going forward. We pooled resources, we joined forces, we united our efforts. I cannot say enough about Matthew. He has been always cheerful, never intimidating. His editing gift can disentangle in moments, clear and move the story, all the while considering the connection and parallel history between Pierre and the Mayo brothers.

I watched as Mayo professionals designed, illustrated and developed my manuscript, made richer with Matthew's care and Mayo research.

I have gone from following the stars to magic to a miracle. If only I could tell Pierre, and my father.

I am blessed to emerge from the process content, cheerful, relaxed, healthy, warm in my relationship with Mayo Clinic Press. I can verify that the culture we see from the outside of the Mayo Clinic is real, and every day I am grateful I was chosen to be part of this team.

We all celebrate *When Winter Came*. The book you hold is what I saw when I was four years old, sitting on Grandpa's knee, peeking into his lockbox and listening to his story.

Nothing has changed.

Acknowledgments

Matthew D. Dacy, M.A., editor

In the Mayo Clinic tradition of teamwork, it is a pleasure to thank those who shared the journey to publish this book.

Working with the author, Mary Beth Sartor Obermeyer, has been a delight. Beth is a consummate storyteller whose email messages and telephone conversations opened new dimensions of the compelling story she wrote. Beth sets the gold standard in her passion and diligence for preserving and sharing her family history. I hope many readers will be inspired by her example in capturing their own family stories.

John T. and Lillian G. Mathews, loyal Mayo Clinic patients and benefactors, provide friendship and encouragement along with vital philanthropic support. This book continues their advocacy for communicating our institutional history and culture, which began with the founding of Mayo Clinic Heritage Hall and the Mayo Clinic Heritage Film Series in 2004.

I am grateful to subject matter specialists who reviewed the text, shared their knowledge and offered key collaborations. Gregory A. Poland, M.D., wrote the welcome message that begins this book, connecting the values and efforts of Pierre Sartor, M.D., a century ago with the issues of our time. Christopher J. Boes, M.D., reviewed the text and coauthored the essay that

315

links Dr. Sartor with Mayo Clinic. Kerry D. Olsen, M.D., provided valuable information about the probable cause of Pierre Sartor's childhood hearing ailment and contemporary methods of treatment. W. Bruce Fye, M.D., offered significant commentary and suggestions, particularly about the early institutional history of Mayo Clinic and the academic milieu of Pierre's medical education. Anne D. Brataas, M.S., researched and compiled information on influenza and the 1918-1919 pandemic; she also graciously shared her professional assessments of the work of Edward C. Rosenow, M.D., whose serum figures in Dr. Sartor's memoir. Brooke A. Weber, Ph.D., located important information including census records and archival images. Thanks to Adam C. Briggs, J.D.; Erika A. Riggin, M.L.S.; Katherine J. Warner, M.L.S., Shari Chertok; and Nancy Kern for expertise in policy and securing permission for reprinting content.

Mayo Clinic Press assembled a stellar team whose wisdom and expertise bring the words of Beth's story to life. Thanks to Daniel J. Harke, M.B.A., publisher; Nina E. Wiener, editor-in-chief; Karen R. Wallevand, M.S., senior editor; Stewart (Jay) J. Koski, M.F.A., art director; Darren L. Wendt, designer; James E. Rownd, illustrator; Paul Flessland, photographer; and Kelly L. Hahn in marketing. Christine N. Boyer, associate product manager, collaborated with the author in many ways, including the safe transportation of Sartor family artifacts to and from photo sessions at Mayo Clinic.

As in many other projects over many years, Jeanne M. Klein, coordinator of Mayo Clinic Heritage Days, provided skillful project administration and valuable professional judgment.

The W. Bruce Fye Center for the History of Medicine is a treasured repository of Mayo Clinic archives. The staff's expertise and dedication are an inspiration to me and to many others who have the privilege of collaborating with them. Thanks to Renee E. Ziemer, coordinator, and her team: Nicole L. Babcock, Emily J. Christopherson, Karen F. Koka and Mona K. Stevermer.

The Sisters of St. Francis are central to the story of Mayo Clinic, particularly during the period covered in this book. I appreciate the support of Sister Lauren Weinandt, archivist of the Saint Marys Campus of Mayo Clinic Hospital-Rochester, and Sister Marisa McDonald, archivist of the Academy of Our Lady of Lourdes at Assisi Heights, the sisters' congregational home in Rochester, Minnesota.

Exploring the medical education of Pierre and Guido Sartor brought connections to archival specialists at other institutions. Thanks to Kathryn Young, M.L.S., Loyola University Chicago, and to the staff of Registrar Services, University of Iowa.

Before medical school, Guido Sartor attended Columbia College in Dubuque, Iowa, known today as Loras College, which by coincidence is the undergraduate alma mater of my youngest daughter, Gina M. Haze. I am grateful to our family's friend, President James E. Collins, who referred me to Heidi Pettit, access services and special collections librarian, for information on Guido's academic experience there. Thanks, also, to Luke Pattarozzi, assistant director of marketing for enrollment, who provided a timeline of Loras College history.

I have worked with three supervisors in the Department of Development during the life of this project, each of whom expressed ongoing interest and support. Thanks to Alaine M. Westra, Melissa A. Gerlesberger and Carla J. Tentis. Our department is blessed with administrative assistant colleagues whose helpfulness and good cheer make every interaction a pleasure. Thanks to Jennifer C. Conrad, Patricia J. Tupper, Sarah F. Langenfeld, Hannah S. Friedrich and Alyssa M. Waters.

Permit me to conclude these acknowledgments with the person I sought out at the start of the project: my wife, Lea C. Dacy. Lea's support sustains me in all things, and her writing and editing skills were particularly important as I worked on this manuscript. In addition, she allowed our dining room to become mission command of *When Winter Came* for nearly two years. Lea, I believe that Mary Magdalene Winandy Sartor, who let her husband convert their kitchen into an operating room, is smiling upon you!

317

Family Trees

LUXEMBOURG

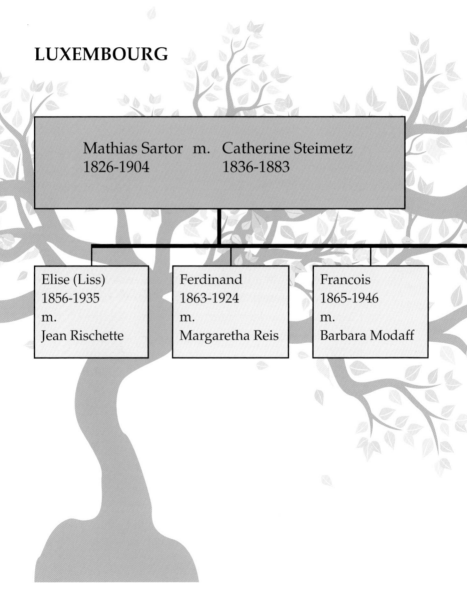

Mathias Sartor m. Catherine Steimetz
1826-1904   1836-1883

Elise (Liss)
1856-1935
m.
Jean Rischette

Ferdinand
1863-1924
m.
Margaretha Reis

Francois
1865-1946
m.
Barbara Modaff

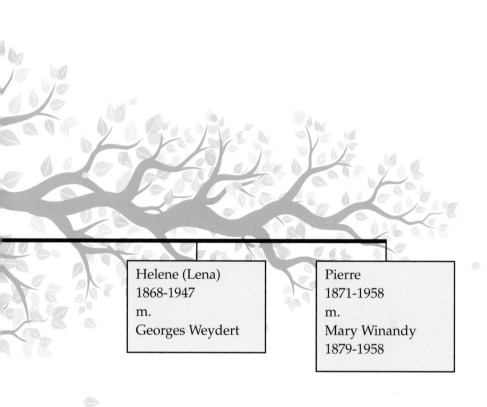

Helene (Lena)
1868-1947
m.
Georges Weydert

Pierre
1871-1958
m.
Mary Winandy
1879-1958

CHICAGO

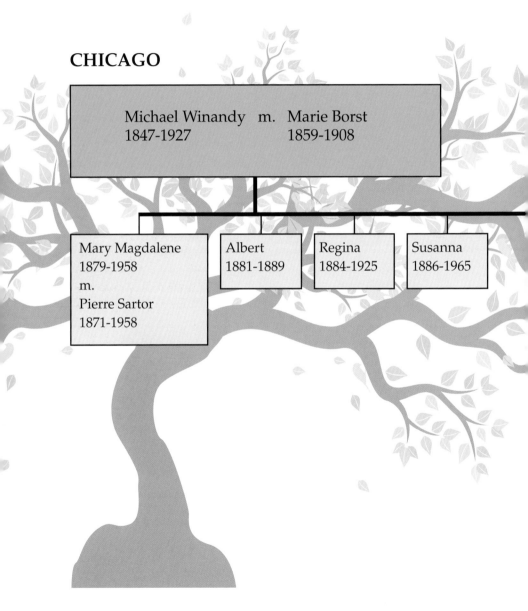

Michael Winandy m. Marie Borst
1847-1927 1859-1908

Mary Magdalene
1879-1958
m.
Pierre Sartor
1871-1958

Albert
1881-1889

Regina
1884-1925

Susanna
1886-1965

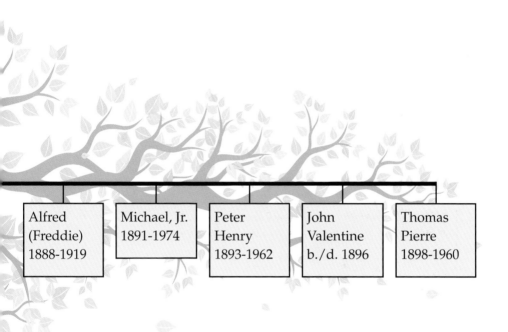

Alfred (Freddie) 1888-1919

Michael, Jr. 1891-1974

Peter Henry 1893-1962

John Valentine b./d. 1896

Thomas Pierre 1898-1960

IOWA

Pierre Sartor m. Mary Magdalene Winandy
1871-1958   1879-1958

Mary Catherine
(May)
1899-1985

Magdalene
1902-1979

Guido
1906-2004
m.
Luella Recker
1909-1995

Celeste
b. 1932

Mary Elizabeth
(Mary Beth)
b. 1942
m.
Thomas Obermeyer
1941-2014

Julie
1949-2007

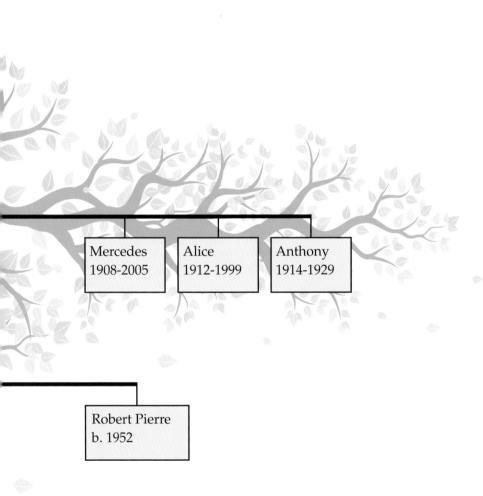

Mercedes
1908-2005

Alice
1912-1999

Anthony
1914-1929

Robert Pierre
b. 1952

Endnotes

Works that are referenced once or a few times are included in specific endnotes. Works that are more frequently referenced use author surname or other identifier in the endnotes along with additional information in Principal Works Cited. Thanks to Mayo Clinic and the Sisters of St. Francis for permission to cite archival materials and published sources within their collections and copyrights.

Dr. Sartor and Mayo Clinic: Collaboration and Inspiration

- Mayo Clinic Model of Care: *https://history.mayoclinic.org/ toolkit/mayo-clinic-model-of-care.php.*
- The vision and determination of Mother Alfred Moes to build Saint Marys Hospital has been told in multiple books, films and other media. For example, see Whelan, Vol. I, pp. 43-52.
- The origin of the name "Mayo Clinic" and distinctive attributes of the institution are described in Fye, pp. 39-41.
- Dr. William J. Mayo's statement about "the glory of medicine" is quoted in Willius, p. 75.
- ". . . spread like wildfire . . ." Pierre Sartor, "Thrills of My Life," p. III.
- "All in all, the community of Titonka . . ." Letter from A.

O. Mardorf, April 8, 1952; author's collection.

- Pierre Sartor used the phrases "nothing easy" and "keep agoing" in his writing and conversation. On p. VIII of "Thrills of My Life," he wrote that he had no fire to warm his office in the winter of 1918: "nobody to keep it agoing."

INTRODUCTION

- General, historical and cultural information about Luxembourg is from *https://www.visitluxembourg.com/*.
- "Right here let me say . . ." Pierre Sartor, "Thrills of My Life," p. VII.
- David Brooks, *The Road to Character*. Random House Trade Paperback Edition, 2016; p. 21.

CHAPTER 1

- "Monday morning when we awoke . . ." *Titonka Topic*, February 6, 1919.
- ". . . came down with the flu . . ." Pierre Sartor, "Thrills of My Life," p. XII.
- "My heart break," a term that Pierre Sartor used conversationally, is a colloquial form of "My heart breaks" and expressed his sadness at a situation.
- ". . . one of my rules strictly enforced . . ." Pierre Sartor, "Thrills of My Life," p. IX.
- *The Secret Garden* by Frances Hodgson Burnett was first published in the U.S. in book form in 1911 by the Frederick A. Stokes Company.

CHAPTER 2

- For a history of "the slough" ("slew") and its current management by the U.S. Fish and Wildlife Service as the Union Slough National Wildlife Refuge, see *https://www.fws.gov/refuge/union-slough*.
- Pierre Sartor told the story of caring for the sick child in

"Thrills of My Life," pp. XII-XIII.

CHAPTER 3

- There are multiple printed, online and video information sources about Whit Tuesday in Luxembourg, the Hopping Procession and the Legend of the Fiddler Thief. For example, see "Echternach Hopping Procession" in *https://luxembourg.public.lu/en/society-and-culture/festivals-and-traditions/echternach-hopping-procession.html*. See also "Hopping Procession of Echternach in United Nations Educational, Scientific and Cultural Organization (UNESCO) Intangible Cultural Heritage: *https://ich.unesco.org/en/RL/hopping-procession-of-echternach-00392*.
- *Hans Brinker; or, the Silver Skates: A Story of Life in Holland* is a novel by Mary Mapes Dodge, published in 1865 by James O'Kane.
- The proverb "Har ass Har . . ." was quoted in a letter dated January 31, 1948, to Pierre Sartor from Emile Weydert, his nephew, who lived in Luxembourg. The letter was published in the *Titonka Topic* on February 19, 1948.

CHAPTER 4

- Robert J. Casey, *The Land of Haunted Castles*. The Century Co., 1921.
- There are multiple versions of prayers for, by and about physicians, representing a variety of time periods and faith traditions. The author's collection includes a copy of the Physician's Prayer owned by Pierre Sartor. In *A Grandparent's Book*, p. 86, Guido Sartor listed the Physician's Prayer as his favorite prayer.
- Description of chronic serous otitis media summarized from email from Kerry D. Olsen, M.D., to Matthew D. Dacy, March 10, 2021, and January 3, 2022. See also "The History of Myringotomy and Grommets" by Joanne Rimmer, M.A., et al. in *Ear, Nose & Throat Journal*, 2020,

Vol. 99 (IS) 2S-7S. *https://journals.sagepub.com/ doi/10.1177/0145561320914438*. For a contemporary description of the condition, see "Ear Infection" published by Mayo Clinic in *https://www.mayoclinic.org/diseases-conditions/ear-infections/symptoms-causes/syc-20351616*.

- "We always . . . looked upon Doctor Sartor as a very kind doctor." Letter from A.O. Mardorf, April 8, 1952; author's collection.

- "I perfectly recollect your name," along with descriptions of Pierre while studying in Echternach, are from a letter to Pierre Sartor from Rev. Peter Trierweiler, his former schoolmate; undated but associated with Pierre's trip to see Rev. Trierweiler, which was reported in the *Titonka Topic*, September 5, 1952; author's collection.

- Pierre's academic records from Luxembourg, circa 1880s-1893; author's collection.

- For historical context of Pierre's education before medical school in the United States, see "History of Education in Luxembourg" published in K12 Academics by Easton (Connecticut) Country Day School: *https://www.k12academics.com/Education%20Worldwide/Education%20in%20 Luxembourg/history-education-luxembourg#:~:text=The%20 history%20of%20education%20in,education%20courses%20 for%20a%20while*.

- Information about Rev. Nicolas Moes is from email from Lucien Wagner to the author, March 8, 2021, and January 2, 2022.

- For information about Mother Alfred Moes, see Whelan, Vol. I, pp. 19-56.

- Original 1893 letters from Ferdinand Sartor in the United States to Pierre Sartor in Luxembourg, written in German, and a 1980s translation into English by Emile Weydert, Pierre's nephew; author's collection.

- Panic of 1893: "Banking Panics of the Gilded Age: 1863-1913" by Gary Richardson and Tim Sablik in Federal Reserve History: *https://www.federalreservehistory.org/ essays/banking-panics-of-the-gilded-age*.

CHAPTER 5

- For information on RMS *Lucania*, see "Lucania Luxury" in National Museums Liverpool: *https://www.liverpoolmuseums.org.uk/stories/lucania-luxury*.

CHAPTER 6

- "The facilities of this institution . . ." comes from "Bennett Medical College and Hospital," no publisher or date; author's collection.
- For information on the Chicago church that the Winandy and Sartor families attended, see "St. Henry Church," published by Rogers Park / West Ridge Historical Society: *https://rpwrhs.org/w/index.php?title=St._Henry_Church*.
- For information about the World's Fair, see Donald L. Miller, *City of the Century: The Epic of Chicago and the Making of America*; Simon & Schuster trade paperback edition, 2003; pp. 488-532.
- "The Trolley Song" (from *Meet Me in St. Louis*)
  Words and Music by Hugh Martin and Ralph Blane
  © 1943 (Renewed) METRO-GOLDWYN-MAYER INC.
  © 1944 (Renewed) EMI FEIST CATALOG INC.
  All Rights Controlled by EMI FEIST CATALOG INC.
  (Publishing) and ALFRED MUSIC (Print)
  All Rights Reserved
  Used by Permission of ALFRED MUSIC
- Information about Chicago is from Miller, pp. 16-17.
- "City of the Big Shoulders" comes from the poem "Chicago" by Carl Sandburg; first published in *Poetry: A Magazine of Verse*; Vol. III, no. vi, March 1914.
- Information about Buffalo Bill (William Frederick Cody) comes from "Buffalo Bill: American Showman" by Joseph J. Di Certo. Encyclopaedia Britannica: *https://www.britannica.com/biography/William-F-Cody*.
- Information about Annie Oakley (Phoebe Ann Mosey) comes from "Annie Oakley," Buffalo Bill Center of the

West: *https://centerofthewest.org/explore/buffalo-bill/research/annie-oakley/*.

- Information on Frederick Jackson Turner, Ph.D., comes from "Frederick Jackson Turner: American Historian" by John Faragher. Encyclopaedia Britannica: *https://www.britannica.com/biography/Frederick-Jackson-Turner*.
- The Mayo brothers attended the 1893 Chicago World's Fair. See Whelan, Vol. I, p. 64.

CHAPTER 7

- Information on Louis Pasteur is from "Louis Pasteur: French Chemist and Microbiologist" by Agnes Ullmann. Encyclopaedia Britannica: *https://www.britannica.com/biography/Louis-Pasteur*.
- Information on Wilhelm Conrad Röntgen comes from "Wilhelm Conrad Röntgen: German Physicist" by the Editors of Encyclopaedia Britannica: *https://www.britannica.com/biography/Wilhelm-Rontgen*.
- Description of Bennett College of Eclectic Medicine and Surgery is from "History of Bennett" in *EmDee*. Published by The Junior Class of Bennett Medical College, Medical Department of Loyola University, Chicago, Illinois, 1916; p. 11. Archives & Special Collections, Loyola University Chicago, Cudahay Library — Lake Shore Campus.
- For information about trends in medical education in the late 19th century, see "Medical Education" in Encyclopedia.com: *https://www.encyclopedia.com/history/united-states-and-canada/us-history/medical-education*.
- For information about Chicago's experience with 19th-century medical education, including the participation of women and African Americans, see "Medical Education" in Encyclopedia of Chicago: *http://www.encyclopedia.chicagohistory.org/pages/805.html*.
- The significance of Abraham Flexner's 1910 report, "Medical Education in the United States and Canada," which was sponsored by the Carnegie Foundation for the

Advancement of Teaching, is covered in Fye, pp. 46-47. The critical assessment of Bennett Medical College is described in Matré, p. 11.

- For information on how Bennett Medical College became part of Loyola University, see Matré, pp. 10-17; "History of Bennett" in *EmDee*, p. 11; and Encyclopedia of Chicago: *http://www.encyclopedia.chicagohistory.org/pages/805.html*.
- "Miss M.E. Bliss, M.D." was recognized as having the highest grades in Pierre's class in *The Chicago Medical Times*, Vol. 29, April 1896, p. 187.
- For information on the United States Supreme Court Case Plessy v. Ferguson, see National Archives Milestone Documents: Plessy v. Ferguson: *https://www.archives.gov/milestone-documents/plessy-v-ferguson*.
- For information on Dr. John Dill Robertson, see Matré, pp. 12-14 and Dr. Robertson's obituary in the *New York Times*, August 21, 1931, p. 11.
- Loyola University's tribute to Dr. John Dill Robertson is quoted in Matré, p. 14.
- "On the Street Where You Live" is a song by Frederick Loewe and Alan Jay Lerner from *My Fair Lady* (1956).

CHAPTER 8

- Information about Pierre's medical school graduation comes from *The Chicago Medical Times*, Vol. 29, April 1896, pp. 187-191. Invitation to the graduation and related items are in the author's collection.
- Pierre was described as "one of the best" in his class in *The Chicago Medical Times*, Vol. 29, October 1896, p. 393.
- "Sporting a sweeping black mustache . . ." For this description of Pierre's arrival in Bancroft, Iowa, see "Titonka Doctor is 'Iowa's General Practitioner of 1953'" by Bob Spiegel in the *Des Moines Tribune*, April 29, 1953, p. 3.
- Information about Bancroft can be found in "Bancroft, Iowa": *https://www.bancroftiowa.com/about*.
- For information on Kossuth County, see "History of

Kossuth County, Iowa," published by Kossuth County Economic Development Corporation: *https://kossuth-edc.com/county-community/history-of-kossuth/.*

- "Ya Got Trouble" is a song by Meredith Willson from *The Music Man*, which premiered in 1957.
- The story of Dr. Robert Cogley is found in "The Medical History of Kossuth County" by Charles Henry Cretzmeyer, M.D. in *Journal of Iowa State Medical Society*, January 1958, Vol. XLVIII, No. 1, pp. 43.
- Pierre's journal and other artifacts, including his reference to "19-lb. baby" are in the author's collection.
- Mary Winandy's First Communion book: author's collection.
- "American Century." See "Milestones 1937-1941: Henry Luce and 20th Century U.S. Internationalism" in the United States Department of State, Office of the Historian: *https://history.state.gov/milestones/1937-1945/internationalism.*
- For a description of Alençon Lace, see "Craftsmanship of Alençon needle lace-making" in United Nations Educational, Scientific and Cultural Organization (UNESCO) Intangible Cultural Heritage: *https://ich.unesco.org/en/RL/craftsmanship-of-alenon-needle-lace-making-00438.*
- A description of Marshall Field's is found in Miller, pp. 254-273. See also "Marshall Field's [The Great Clocks — by Graham, Anderson, Probst and White]." Chicago Architecture and Cityscape, January 2, 2009: *http://chicago-architecture-jyoti.blogspot.com/2009/01/great-clock.html.*

CHAPTER 9

- "Iowa Stubborn"
Words and Music by Meredith Willson
© 1957 (Renewed) Frank Music Corp. and Meredith Willson Music, LLC
Administered by MPL Music Publishing, Inc.
All Rights Reserved. International Copyright Secured.
Reprinted by Permission of Hal Leonard LLC
- For a history of St. John the Baptist Church and its parish

school, see "St. John Parish" in *https://bggoldenbears.org/about/parishes/bancroft.html*. See also "St. John the Baptist Church" on the website for Bancroft, Iowa: *https://www.bancroftiowa.com/index.asp?SEC=542D73A7-10CB-4377-9A1E-B44C9E940C6D&DE=233BAAAE-B53D-4886-BC07-A56776506315.*

CHAPTER 10

- "He was as cheerful a neighbor as I remember having. …" Letter from Donald H. James, undated; author's collection.
- The injury of "Little Miss Ida May" was published in the *Algona Courier* on November 1, 1907.
- "I think one of Dr. Sartor's secrets . . ." Letter from Donald H. James, undated; author's collection.
- Pierre Sartor's efforts to fumigate and disinfect local houses were reported by the Board of Health in the *Titonka Topic* on April 2, 1908.
- Information on Walter Reed is from "Walter Reed: American Pathologist and Bacteriologist" by E. Ashworth Underwood. Encyclopedia Brittanica: *https://www.britannica.com/biography/Walter-Reed*.
- "I could diagnose." Pierre Sartor, "Thrills of My Life," p. I.
- Description of Dr. William Worrall Mayo as having a "questing spirit" is from Mayo, p. 5; "he was a perfectionist . . ." is from p. 16.
- For Dr. William J. Mayo's description of how he and his brother, Dr. Charles H. Mayo, served as "moral custodians" of "the people's money" and returned it to the public in the form of advanced medical education and research, see Willius, p. 106.
- Many books about the history of Mayo Clinic include descriptions of the 1883 tornado. For example, see Clapesattle, pp. 242-245 and Whelan, Vol. I, pp. 39-42.
- "With our faith and hope and energy, it will succeed" is included in many histories of Mayo Clinic. For example, see Whelan, Vol. I, p. 44.

- "The people of the community also admired another quality of the good doctor . . ." Letter from A.O. Mardorf, April 8, 1952; author's collection.
- Pierre's treatment of Cecilia Grandjennet and affirmation by the Mayo brothers was published in the *Algona Courier*, November 1, 1907.
- Pierre's signature in the Mayo guest book on February 3, 1908: Mayo Clinic Archives of the W. Bruce Fye Center for the History of Medicine.
- "The rush of medical visitors" to Rochester, Minnesota, as described in *Canada Lancet* is quoted in Clapesattle, p. 452.
- The doctor from St. Louis who wrote "Among the many physicians who visit the Mayos . . ." is quoted in Clapesattle, p. 449.
- "There was as much to be heard as seen . . ." comes from Clapesattle, p. 453.
- "Both men were perfectly frank . . . ." Clapesattle, p. 457.
- Pierre's treatment of Mrs. J.M. McCowien was published in the *Algona Courier*, November 1, 1907.
- For the description of Dr. Charles W. Mayo's "medically-saturated upbringing" in which "almost every adult male in our family was a doctor . . . ," see Mayo, p. 1.
- Dr. William D. Haggard, a friend and colleague of the Mayos, described Dr. Will and Dr. Charlie as "the surgical travelers of the world." See Clapesattle, p. 681.
- The Mayowood greenhouses and annual Mayowood Chrysanthemum Show are described in Clapesattle, p. 694.
- "Visitors who were shown through the Mayowood greenhouses were always astonished . . ." Clapesattle, p. 475.
- The *Titonka Topic* reported on September 15, 1927, that S.B. French visited Mayo Clinic. The story of the Heetland family was published on February 6, 1930.
- The origin of the name "Mayo Clinic" is described in Fye, pp. 39-41.
- Dr. William J. Mayo's explanation that the name of Mayo Clinic "was given to us by our friends" is quoted in Fye, p. 41.

CHAPTER 11

- For a history of the song "Home on the Range," see Song of America: *https://songofamerica.net/song/home-on-the-range/*.
- Walter Lord, *The Good Years: From 1900 to the First World War.* Harper and Brothers, 1960.
- Information about the Sartor household in the 1910 Census: "Rosalie [illegible]," enumeration district 160, page 3B, line 77. Accessed via Ancestry.com. *1910 United States Federal Census* [database online]. Lehi, UT, USA: Ancestry.com Operations Inc., 2006.

CHAPTER 12

- Dr. William J. Mayo's statement that medical science has no country is quoted in Clapesattle, p. 572.
- For information about how a German official described the treaty guaranteeing Belgian neutrality as a "scrap of paper," see *https://www.firstworldwar.com/source/scrapofpaper2.htm*.
- For information on Grand Duchess Marie-Adélaïde and the experience of Luxembourg during World War I, see *https://windowstoworldhistory.weebly.com/grand-duchess-marie-adelaide-of-luxembourg-is-a-symbol-of-effective-rule.html* and "Occupation of Luxembourg" by Richard Seiwerath in Encyclopedia of the First World War: *https://encyclopedia.1914-1918-online.net/article/occupation_of_luxembourg*.
- For information on the German invasion and occupation of Belgium during World War I, see "Remember Belgium" in Army Heritage Center Foundation *https://www.armyheritage.org/soldier-stories-information/remember-belgium/*.
- For information about Evan Jones, a passenger from Ottumwa, Iowa, who died in the sinking of the RMS *Lusitania*, see *https://www.rmslusitania.info/people/third-class/evan-jones/*.
- "Do Your Bit" was a popular phrase during World War I,

which encouraged civilians to support the war effort. See "Docs Teach" from the National Archives: *https://www. docsteach.org/documents/document/little-americans-do-your- bit*. The phrase was modified for various wartime purpos- es. For example, Mary Sartor and her friends rallied to the exhortation, "Knit Your Bit."

- Pierre Sartor's application for the Medical Reserves Corps of the U.S. Army; author's collection.
- *Over the Top: By An American Soldier Who Went* by Arthur Guy Empey was published by A.L. Burt in 1917; the song, "I want to go home," is on p. 233. The book was serialized in many newspapers, including the *Titonka Topic* from May 2 to October 31, 1918.
- Mary Sartor's recipe card; author's collection.

CHAPTER 13

- For information about Dr. Robert M. Wallace, see "The Medical History of Kossuth County" by Charles Henry Cretzmeyer, M.D., in *Journal of Iowa State Medical Society*, January 1958, Vol. XLVIII, No. 1, pp. 48 and 49. On Febru- ary 14, 1918, the *Titonka Topic* reported that Dr. Wallace had sold his practice to Dr. Pierre Sartor.
- The origin of the 1918 influenza pandemic is described in Barry, pp. 91-97.

CHAPTER 14

- For a history of Titonka and meaning of the name, see the home page of the City of Titonka: *https://titonka.com/*.
- The population of Titonka in 1910 (278) and 1920 (418) was published in *Fourteenth Census of the United States: 1920 Bulletin; Population: Iowa; Number of Inhabitants by Counties and Minor Civil Division*s. Department of Com- merce, Bureau of the Census, Samuel L. Rogers, Director, p. 23. *https://www2.census.gov/library/publications/decennial/ 1920/bulletins/demographics/population-ia-number-of-*

inhabitants.pdf.

- The Lakota and Dakota word "tatanka" for "buffalo" is used in the film *Dances with Wolves*. See *Dances with Wolves: The Illustrated Story of the Epic Film* by Kevin Costner, Michael Blake and Jim Wilson. Newmarket Press, 1990, p. 56. In this reference, the word is transliterated as "tatonka."
- "Physicians and the Automobile" by Charles H. Mayo in the *Journal of the American Medical Association*, 1901, Vol. 36, p. 1002.
- "A car run by foot pedals." Guido Sartor, *A Grandparent's Book*, p. 15.
- "Learned [to drive] at 12 years." Guido Sartor, *A Grandparent's Book*, p. 32.
- "Good Roads and the Mayo Brothers." Clark W. Nelson, *Mayo Roots: Profiling the Origins of Mayo Clinic*. Mayo Foundation for Medical Education and Research, 1990, pp. 86-87.
- For information on travel in Iowa during this period, see *Approaching the Turn of the Century: Discovering Historic Iowa Transportation Milestones*, published by the Iowa Department of Transportation, Director's Staff Division, February 1999: *https://iowadot.gov/histbook.pdf.* For a description of the "Red Ball" route, see "Early Road Markings," p. 11; "Tourist Road Routes," p. 17; and "Impact of World War I," p. 20.
- The outbreak of influenza at Camp Funston in March 1918 is described in Barry, pp. 95-97.
- Dr. Loring Miner's report of "influenza of severe type," which was published in *Public Health Reports,* is described in Barry, pp. 94-95.
- Origin of the term "Spanish flu," which misidentified the location of its outbreak, is described in Barry, p. 171.
- The three waves of influenza and fatalities in the U.S and around the world are described in "1918 Pandemic Influenza Historic Timeline," published by Centers for Disease Control and Prevention: *https://www.cdc.gov/flu/pandemic-*

resources/1918-commemoration/pandemic-timeline-1918.htm.

- For a report of U.S. combat deaths in World War I (53,402), see "War Losses (USA)" by Carol S. Byerly in Encyclopedia of the First World War: *https://encyclopedia.1914-1918-online.net/article/war_losses_usa.*
- The loss of more than 6,000 people in Iowa to the influenza pandemic is cited in many sources. For example, see "Lessons for Iowa from the Spanish Flu Pandemic of 1918" by Steffen Schmidt in *The Gazette* (Cedar Rapids, Iowa): *https://www.thegazette.com/guest-columnists/lessons-for-iowa-from-the-spanish-flu-pandemic-of-1918/.*

CHAPTER 15

- "Summer over. Fall season here." Pierre Sartor, "Thrills of My Life," p. I.
- "He was hardly more than five feet, four inches . . ." This description of Hercule Poirot comes from *The Mysterious Affair at Styles: A Detective Story* by Agatha Christie, published by Dodd, Mead and Company, 1920, p. 35.
- "The little grey cells" is a phrase in *The A.B.C. Murders*, a novel by Agatha Christie, published by Dodd, Mead and Company in 1936; the phrase "order, method" comes from a short story by Agatha Christie entitled "The Adventure of 'The Western Star,'" first published in 1923 in a periodical entitled *The Sketch.* Both phrases are cited in *Little Grey Cells: The Quotable Poirot,* edited by David Brawn. HarperCollins Publishers, 2015.
- The story of the Isolation Unit is told in many histories of Saint Marys Hospital. See Clapesattle, pp. 569-570. See Whelan, Vol. I, pp. 104-105.
- Arrival of the first patient in the Isolation Unit: *Annals of Saint Marys Hospital*, p. 109.
- For information about Union Slough National Wildlife Refuge, see *https://www.fws.gov/refuge/union-slough.*
- The account of Billy Johnson accidentally shooting a hunter was covered in the *Titonka Topic* on September 26, 1918.

- Bub Ribsamen was a friend of Guido Sartor; they were part of a group of young men who were interested in cars and radios. The author's collection includes a period photo of Bub Ribsamen.
- For information about 4-H activities that Pierre and Mary's children would have engaged in during the World War I era, see Iowa 4-H Foundation, "Kossuth County, Iowa 4-H History." *https://www.iowa4hfoundation.org/index.cfm/36964/4060/kossuth_county_4h_history*.
- For information about Chicago's experience with the influenza pandemic and the role of Dr. John Dill Robertson, see "Chicago, Illinois" in Influenza Encyclopedia / The American Influenza Epidemic of 1918-1919: A Digital Encyclopedia, published by the University of Michigan Center for the History of Medicine and Michigan Publishing, University of Michigan Library: *http://www.influenzaarchive.org/cities/city-chicago.html*. See also "How Chicago Dealt with the 1918 Spanish Flu" by Edward McClelland, *Chicago Magazine*, March 17, 2020: *https://www.chicagomag.com/city-life/march-2020/how-chicago-dealt-with-the-1918-spanish-flu/*.
- The description of doctors in Chicago who saw 60 to 90 patients per day during the pandemic is from Morris Fishbein, *Morris Fishbein, M.D., An Autobiography*. Doubleday and Co., 1969, p. 70.
- "'My God,' I was a-thinking …." and "Traveling salesmen telling stories of flu …" are from Pierre Sartor, "Thrills of My Life," p. I.

CHAPTER 16

- "Then — on the first of October . . . " Pierre's description of the arrival of influenza in Titonka and his care of his first patient with the condition comes from "Thrills of My Life," pp. I-II.
- The Centers for Disease Control and Prevention describes the spike in fatalities from influenza in October 1918 in

https://www.cdc.gov/flu/pandemic-resources/1918-commemoration/1918-pandemic-history.htm.

- "Rock Island Line" is an American folk song whose roots date to the late 1920s and which has been recorded by many musicians, often with variations to the lyrics. See "The Rock Island Line is the Road to Ride" in *The Music Court*: *https://musiccourtblog.com/2011/09/07/the-rock-island-line-is-the-road-to-ride/.*

- "The successive developments in transportation have been essential in the Mayo rise . . ." Clapesattle, p. 348.

- For a history of the Klondike Mines Railway, see Yukon Nuggets: "The Klondike Mines Railway." *https://yukon-nuggets.com/stories/the-klondike-mines-railway.*

- Information about George Lewis Lamoreux (1886-1960); his mother, Jennie Isenberger Lamoreux ("Grandma L.," 1854-1931); his wife, Myrtle Harriet Plumb Lamoreux ("Mrs. George Lamoreux," 1892-1983) and his wife's brother, Clifford Cyrus Plumb (1896-1951):

    *1910 U.S. Census, Iowa, population schedule. Accessed via Ancestry.com. 1910 United States Federal Census [database online]. Lehi, UT, USA: Ancestry.com Operations Inc., 2006.

    *1920 U.S. Census, Iowa, population schedule. Accessed via Ancestry.com. 1920 United States Federal Census [database online]. Provo, UT, USA: Ancestry.com Operations, Inc., 2010.

    *Ancestry.com. Iowa, U.S., Death Records, 1880-1904, 1921-1952 [database online]. Lehi, UT, USA: Ancestry.com Operations, Inc., 2017.

    *Ancestry.com. U.S., World War I Draft Registration Cards, 1917-1918 [database online]. Provo, UT, USA: Ancestry.com Operations Inc., 2005.

    *FamilySearch. United States, Veterans Administration Master Index, 1917-1940, database. *https://familysearch.org/ark:/61903/1:1:W9HD-GYT2.*

    *Find A Grave, database. *http://www.findagrave.com.*

    *Joseph A. Whitacre and W.J. Moore, *Marshall County*

in the World War, 1917-1918: A pictorial history of the community's participation in all wartime activities with a complete roster of soldiers and sailors in service, published by Joseph A. Whitacre and W. J. Moore, 1919, pp. 206, 263.

- Pierre's rule, "Windows open" and use of liner shutters, is from "Thrills of My Life," p. IX.
- For a history of Naval Station Great Lakes, its experience in World War I and the influenza pandemic, as well as the music of John Philip Sousa's Bluejacket Band, see *https:// cnrma.cnic.navy.mil/Installations/NAVSTA-Great-Lakes/ About/History/*.
- "The Village Blacksmith" is a poem by Henry Wadsworth Longfellow, first published in 1840. It describes a man who is strong, humble and self-sufficient, balancing his work with his commitment to his family and his role in the community. This image served as a role model for many men in Pierre's and Guido Sartor's generations.
- "George Lamoreux called up Tuesday …" was reported in the *Titonka Topic*, October 31, 1918.
- "The campus is now under strict military police security" is a paraphrase from content in "University Work to Be Continued Despite Influenza" in *The Daily Iowan*, October 6, 1918, Vol. VXIII; New Series Vol. III, p. 1: *https://dailyio-wan.lib.uiowa.edu/DI/1918/di1918-10-06.pdf*.
- Campus conditions at Iowa State College (today, Iowa State University) is described in "A Bird Named Enza Flew to ISU: The Flu Epidemic of 1918" in *Cardinal Tales: The Blog of Special Collections and University Archives at ISU*, January 16, 2015: *https://isuspecialcollections.wordpress. com/2015/01/16/a-bird-named- enza-flew-to-isu-the-flu-epi-demic-of-1918/*.
- The experience of influenza in Iowa is described as an infographic in "The 1918 Flu 100 Years Later," Iowa Department of Health, April 2018: *https://idph.iowa.gov/ Portals/1/userfiles/33/100%20Years%20Infographic%20 Original_final.pdf*.
- "Uncle Sam's Advice on Flu." Serialized article from U.S.

Public Health Service published in the *Titonka Topic*, October 17, 1918.

- "'And then came the flu epidemic!'" Clapesattle, pp. 569-571.
- "The Sisters in charge were in great straits." *Annals of Saint Marys Hospital*, p. 110.
- The appeal for prayers on behalf of the Franciscan Sisters who had influenza (October 21, 1918) is from the Archives of the Rochester Franciscans, Assisi Heights, Rochester, Minnesota.
- "Soon after the Lord sent me the first case . . ." Pierre Sartor, "Thrills of My Life," p. VII.

CHAPTER 17

- Pierre's quotations from "Thrills of My Life" in this chapter: "Somewhere northeast of town . . ." (p. III); "The place was northeast . . ." (pp. III-IV); "In the meantime the Flu spread in town . . ." (p. IV); "Right here, let me mention one of my rules . . ." (p. IX); "One married couple …" (pp. IX-X); "In one farm family . . ." (pp. V-VI); "In another case on the South side of town . . ." (pp. X-XII); and "Doctor Ray in the next town . . ." (pp. VIII-IX).
- As an example of barn dances that were popular at the time, see the announcement of the dance to be held at the Ed Huber barn, published in the *Titonka Topic*, September 26, 1918.
- "As the virulence of the strange disease became better known . . ." *Annals of Saint Marys Hospital*, p. 110.
- The account of Grandma Ringsdorf was published in the *Titonka Topic,* December 12, 1918.
- Two popular songs during the First World War were "Keep the Home-Fires Burning (Till the Boys Come Home)" by Ivor Novello and Lena Guilbert Ford and "Over There" by George M. Cohan.
- Career summary of Dr. Edward C. Rosenow. *Physicians of the Mayo Clinic and the Mayo Foundation*. University of

Minnesota Press, 1937; p. 1197.

- "Dr. Copeland [New York City Health Commissioner] ... was favorably impressed . . ." the *New York Times*, December 13, 1918. p. 9.
- "Dr. Rosenow had an evidence-based, but unproven 'scientific premonition' . . ." email from Anne Brataas to Matthew D. Dacy, April 5, 2021.
- "The day after the *Journal of the American Medical Association* published Dr. Rosenow's offer . . ." Clapesattle, p. 570.
- "Several vaccines, including one developed at the Mayo Clinic . . ." comes from "Epidemic! Iowa Fights the Spanish Flu" by William H. Cumberland in *The Palimpsest*, published by the State Historical Society of Iowa, 62 (1), p. 27.
- "George Lamoreux and family are still down with influenza." *Titonka Topic*, October 17, 1918.
- The statements "Dr. Sartor has had deep respect and confidence from patients of many religious faiths . . . I will never forget the trust and confidence placed in Dr. Sartor by patients who regarded him . . . One of these patients . . ." come from a letter by Donald H. James, undated; author's collection.
- "He has been a doctor of souls as well as a doctor of bodies . . ." Letter from Charles R.J. Quinn, April 7, 1952; author's collection.
- "He was our family doctor when we lived on a mud road far from town . . ." Letter from George and Mona Bonacker, April 9, 1952; author's collection.

CHAPTER 18

- "In the traveling classroom, his horse-drawn buggy . . ." Judith Hartzell, *I Started All This: The Life of Dr. William Worrall Mayo*. Arvi Press, 2004; p. 89.
- The outbreak of influenza, which occurred "suddenly and virulently" at Saint Marys Hospital is described in Clapesattle, p. 569

- The letter from Dr. William J. Mayo describing his brother's illness, December 24, 1918, is quoted in Fye, p. 59.
- The Proclamation by General John Pershing to the people of Luxembourg, November 18, 1918, is quoted in Windows to World History: "Luxembourg's grand Duchess Marie Adelaide Greets General Pershing." *https://windowstoworldhistory.weebly.com/grand-duchess-marie-adelaide-of-luxembourg-is-a-symbol-of-effective-rule.html.*
- Bogus treatments for influenza were legion in the pandemic of 1918-1919. The author recalls Pierre describing many of them. For example, see "11 Bizarre Remedies Used to Treat the 1918 Spanish Flu" by Christopher McFadden, Interesting Engineering, March 9, 2021: *https://interestingengineering.com/11-bizarre-remedies-used-to-treat-the-1918-spanish-flu.* See also "When flu shut down our towns" by Bill Wundram, *Quad City Times*, January 11, 2013, which includes the practice of swallowing a turpentine-soaked cloth tied to a string: *https://qctimes.com/news/opinion/editorial/columnists/bill-wundram/when-flu-shut-down-our-towns/article_e050fc38-5b96-11e2-ab01-0019bb2963f4.html.*
- The *Titonka Topic* reported on local happenings in context of the influenza pandemic on December 12, 1918.
- The illness of Mrs. Hackersbin, who delivered the mail, was published in the *Titonka Topic* on December 26, 1918.
- The motto of U.S. Postal Service is described in "Postal Service Mission and 'Motto.'" Historian, U.S. Postal Service, October 1999: *https://about.usps.com/who/profile/history/pdf/mission-motto.pdf.*
- The *Titonka Topic* described road conditions on December 12, 1918.
- The *Titonka Topic,* June 19, 1919, reported on Pierre and Guido's mishap with getting their car stuck in the mud: "The heaviest downpour of rain that we have ever had in Titonka . . ." and "It evidently was our doctor[']s day for hard luck . . ."
- Pierre's description of how the Model T crank handle

impaled a chicken is paraphrased from family stories and recordings of Pierre sharing his memories.

- "The Last of the Belles" is a short story by F. Scott Fitzgerald, published in *Saturday Evening Post* on March 2, 1929. Reprinted in *The Short Stories of F. Scott Fitzgerald: A New Collection*, edited by Matthew J. Bruccoli. Charles Scribner's Sons, 1989, p. 449.
- "Daddy's Evening Fairy Tale" was published in the *Titonka Topic*, July 25, 1918.
- Description of influenza as a disease that "was little understood" comes from the *Annals of Saint Marys Hospital*, p. 110.
- The statement of St. Francis of Assisi while on his deathbed — "I have done what was mine to do . . ." — is cited in many references. For example, see "St. Francis and the Marrow of the Gospel" by Richard Rohr, OFM, in The Franciscan Spirit Blog, February 4, 2021: *https://www.franciscanmedia.org/franciscan-spirit-blog/st-francis-and-the-marrow-of-the-gospel.*
- The winter's rare blizzard was reported in the *Titonka Topic* on February 6, 1919.
- Charles H. Mayo's statement about the rewards of serving humanity through the practice of medicine is quoted in Willius, p. 24.

CHAPTER 19

- "The Organization and Methods of Contagious Disease Services" by John H. Stokes, M.D., Mayo Clinic, in *Pennsylvania Medical Journal,* August 1919, Vol. 22, pp. 729-736.
- "Thus the epidemic's impact was felt . . ." comes from "Epidemic! Iowa Fights the Spanish Flu" by William H. Cumberland in *The Palimpsest*, published by the State Historical Society of Iowa, 62 (1), p. 29.
- Alfred Winandy's obituary was printed in the *Titonka Topic*, July 10, 1919.
- Pierre's treatment of Fred Boykin, who "stepped on a

rusty nail Monday morning" was published in the *Titonka Topic* on March 25, 1920.

- The experience of W.H. Stott, who fainted in Pierre's office and regained consciousness while Pierre "was pummeling him with his fists" was reported in the *Titonka Topic* on May 13, 1920.

- "My first acquaintance with Dr. Sartor came at the Titonka Lions Club . . ." Letter from Donald H. James, undated; author's collection.

- Pierre's service on the Water Board of the City Council is described in an undated letter from L. (Lester) F. Callies; author's collection.

- Mary Sartor's civic activities were extensively covered in the local press over the years. For example, for the Titonka Women's Club, she reviewed a South American opera and discussed the National Art Gallery (*Mason City Globe Gazette*, November 5, 1942); presented the topic, "News in the Medical World" (*Titonka Topic*, February 12, 1948); and discussed "Our Right to Live" with a special focus on the needs of handicapped children (*Kossuth County Advance*, November 17, 1953).

- "His family has followed his example of community service." Article by Bob Spiegel entitled "Titonka Doctor is 'Iowa's General Practitioner of 1953.'" *Des Moines Tribune*, April 29, 1953, p. 3.

- Guido "drove 400 miles to Chicago when 14 years as only driver." *A Grandparent's Book,* p. 32; author's collection.

- Guido's description of the "garage mechanic who also knew electronics" and encouraged his interest in radio broadcasting comes from *A Grandparent's Book*, p. 34; author's collection.

- "The good doctor has never become wealthy . . ." Letter from G.D. Hart, April 10, 1952; author's collection.

- A photo and description of Guido when he taught in rural schools was published in *History of Riverdale Township, Kossuth County*, p. 80; single page in author's collection. No publisher, no date.

- The description of how Pierre's car broke down in freezing weather while he was driving Guido to his teaching job was reported in the *Titonka Topic*, December 31, 1925.
- "In his blue gardens, men and girls came and went like moths . . ." is from *The Great Gatsby* by F. Scott Fitzgerald. Scribner trade paperback edition, April 2013, p. 39.
- Guido's visit to his "old stomping grounds" was recorded on a family videotape, 1996; author's collection.
- Letter from Guido Sartor to Luella Recker, June 1928, while they were dating; author's collection.
- Luella Sartor's description of teaching the Methodist boys to dance comes from "Life in the Fast Lane," p. 50.
- The *Titonka Topic* published "Anthony Sartor Died Monday Evening" on October 3, 1929.
- Luella Sartor described Guido receiving financial support to attend medical school as "the miracle of our lives" in "Life in the Fast Lane," p. 72.
- Guido and Mary's trip to Mayo Clinic was reported in the *Kossuth County Advance* on August 24, 1930.
- Dr. Charles W. Mayo described the "wretched sense of my own inferiority" in Mayo, pp. 60-61.
- ". . . two can live as cheaply as one . . ." Luella Sartor, "Life in the Fast Lane," p. 72.
- "My Blue Heaven" is a song written by Walter Donaldson and George A. Whiting, published in 1927.
- Luella Sartor described living at her family's farm with baby Celeste while Guido was in medical school in "Life in the Fast Lane," pp. 73-74.
- Pierre's motion to adjourn a meeting of the Kossuth Medical Society in January 1934 during the Great Depression was described in the *Journal of the Iowa State Medical Society*, July 1948, Vol. XLVIII, No. 1, p. 49.
- The story of how Pierre directed the delivery of a baby over the telephone was reported in the *Titonka Topic* on February 13, 1936.
- Description of Pierre as "the typical 'Country Doctor'" comes from a letter from Rev. William Planz, April 9, 1952;

author's collection.

- On August 31, 1939, the *Titonka Topic* reported that "Little Miss Roberta Underbakke" had surgery at Mayo Clinic.
- The train trip by Albert Meyer and his wife — "a patient sufferer for several months" — to Mayo Clinic was covered in the *Titonka Topic* on May 21, 1929.
- Pierre's car trip to Mayo Clinic with four companions was reported in the *Titonka Topic* on May 10, 1938.
- Lee O. Wolfe, editor of the *Titonka Topic*, described his experience at Mayo Clinic on October 14, 1937.
- For information about Luxembourg in World War II, see "Second World War: The Toughest Ordeal for the People" *https://luxembourg.public.lu/en/society-and-culture/history/second-world-war.html.*
- The national motto of Luxembourg is cited in many sources. For example, see *https://www.business-events.lu/articles/post/7-ways-luxembourg-is-totally-unique/.*
- Guido and Luella Sartor's life in Chicago is described in "Life in the Fast Lane," pp. 75-76.
- Luella Sartor described her happiness at moving back to Iowa in "Life in the Fast Lane," p. 76.
- "Dr. Sartor fell on the ice . . . " The *Titonka Topic* reported on this accident on January 25, 1941.
- "I vividly recall how he stayed at the bedside of a member of my family . . ." Letter from A. O. Mardorf, April 8, 1952; author's collection.
- Descriptions of Guido Sartor as a physician, family man, community leader and automobile enthusiast come from the *Mason City Globe Gazette*, February 27, 2004. "Dr. Guido J. Sartor," p. A9, and "'Esteemed' Dr. Sartor dies at 97" by Deb Nicklay, p. A3.

CHAPTER 20

- The *Journal of Iowa State Medical Society* (Vol. 54, no. 6, June 1953, p. 234) quoted Pierre as saying he had "a pretty busy practice."

- "Our offices are but four doors apart . . ." Frank Clark, publisher of the *Titonka Topic*, described Pierre's service on the Chamber of Commerce in a letter dated April 11, 1952; author's collection.
- "After all those years of doctoring and community service . . ." Letter from George and Mary Bonacker, April 9, 1952; author's collection.
- Tape recording of Pierre and Mary's golden anniversary dinner in 1948; author's collection.
- March 30, 1952, was "Dr. Sartor Day" in Titonka, and widely reported in the local press, including the *Algona Advance* on April 3, p. 2.
- On September 19, 1946, the *Titonka Topic* described how Pierre missed the dinner to recognize his 50-year career as a doctor, but received a plaque in his honor later that evening, in a front-page article entitled "Doctor Sartor Honored for 50 Years of Service."
- The Iowa State Medical Society issued a call for letters of endorsement for Pierre's nomination in a letter dated March 26, 1952, from A.B. Phillips, M.D., secretary of the society, to John H. Schutter, M.D., who submitted the nomination; author's collection.
- "It was not done for the love of money nor worldly goods . . ." Letter from Charles R.J. Quinn, April 7, 1952; author's collection.
- Letter from Dr. George Dolmage, May 7, 1953; author's collection.
- On May 10, 1951, the *Titonka Topic* ran a series of tongue-in-cheek blurbs stating "You can complain" about aspects of community life.
- "I am sure that a great many people can say that their life was made a little easier . . ." Letter from Charles R.J. Quinn, April 7, 1952; author's collection.
- The award was announced in the *Des Moines Tribune*, April 29, 1953, p. 3: "Titonka Doctor is 'Iowa's General Practitioner of 1953'" by Bob Spiegel.

- "It was the end of a perfect day for the doctor . . . he wasn't called away to care for a patient." *Algona Advance*, March 29, 1952.
- "The little roly-poly cherub we are gathered here to honor today . . ." is from a typewritten tribute to Pierre by his longtime friend and colleague, Dr. C.R. Cretzmeyer. Handwritten notes on the one-page document indicate that Dr. Cretzmeyer used this introduction on several occasions in the mid-1950s; author's collection.
- *New Horizons: Iowa's Cancer Magazine*, published by the Iowa Division of the American Cancer Society, Mason City, Iowa, featured Pierre on its cover of the fall 1953 issue with an article on p. 2: "Focus on the Iowa Doctor."
- "Mother looked at me . . ." Pierre Sartor, "Thrills of my Life," p, XIII.

CONCLUSION

- *"Don't Believe It!" Says the Doctor*; August A. Thomen, M.D.; with handwritten inscription "To Father" from "G.J. Sartor, M.D.," author's collection
- "Miracle of relationships" is a phrase from Whelan, Vol. II p. 222.

INSIDE BACK COVER

- "He was our family doctor when we lived on a mud road far from town . . ." Letter from George and Mona Bonacker, April 9. 1952; author's collection.
- "The good doctor has never become wealthy . . ." Letter from G.D. Hart, April 10, 1952; author's collection.
- "All in all, the community of Titonka knows that Dr. Sartor is practicing among them to serve them." Letter from A. O. Mardorf, April 8, 1952; author's collection.

Principal Works Cited

- Barry, John M. *The Great Influenza: The Story of the Deadliest Pandemic in History.* Penguin Books, 2018.
- Clapesattle, Helen. *The Doctors Mayo.* University of Minnesota Press, 1941.
- Fye, W. Bruce. *Caring for the Heart: Mayo Clinic and the Rise of Specialization.* Oxford University Press. Mayo Foundation for Medical Education and Research, 2015.
- Matré, Richard A. with Marilu Matré. *Loyola University and Its Medical Center: A Century of Courage and Turmoil: A History of the Stritch College of Medicine and the Chicago College of Dental Surgery at Loyola University of Chicago.* Department of Printing Services, Loyola University Chicago, 1995.
- Mayo, Charles W. *Mayo: The Story of My Family and My Career.* Doubleday, 1969.
- Miller, Donald L. *City of the Century: The Epic of Chicago and the Making of America.* Simon & Schuster trade paperback edition, 2003.
- Obermeyer, Mary Beth Sartor. Family photos, documents and other artifacts from early 19th century to the present. Author's collection.
- Sartor, Guido. Handwritten information, June 28, 1983, in *A Grandparent's Book: Thoughts, Memories, and Hopes for a Grandchild.* Rawson, Wade Publishers, Inc. No date. Author's collection.
- Sartor, Luella. "Life in the Fast Lane." Typed memoir, 1986. Author's collection.

- Sartor, Pierre. "Thrills of my life — specifically, my 'Flu Life.'" Handwritten manuscript; no date, but approximately 1953. Typed transcript, March 3, 2012. Author's collection.
- Sisters of St. Francis. *Annals of Saint Marys Hospital*. Unpublished chronicle, 1889-present. Sisters of St. Francis, Mayo Clinic, Rochester, Minnesota.
- The *Titonka Topic* was a newspaper in Titonka, Iowa, that was published from 1899 to 2017; it provides a wealth of information about the everyday activities of Pierre and his contemporaries. Digital copies of the *Titonka Topic* and other regional newspapers are available at newspaperarchive.com: *https://newspaperarchive.com/*.
- Whelan, Ellen. [Vol. I] *The Sisters' Story: Saint Marys Hospital — Mayo Clinic, 1889 to 1939*. Mayo Foundation for Medical Education and Research, 2002. [Vol. II] *The Sisters' Story: Saint Marys Hospital — Mayo Clinic*, 1939 to 1980. Mayo Foundation for Medical Education and Research, 2007.
- Willius, Fredrick A. *Aphorisms of Dr. Charles Horace Mayo and Dr. William James Mayo*. Mayo Foundation for Medical Education and Research, 1990.

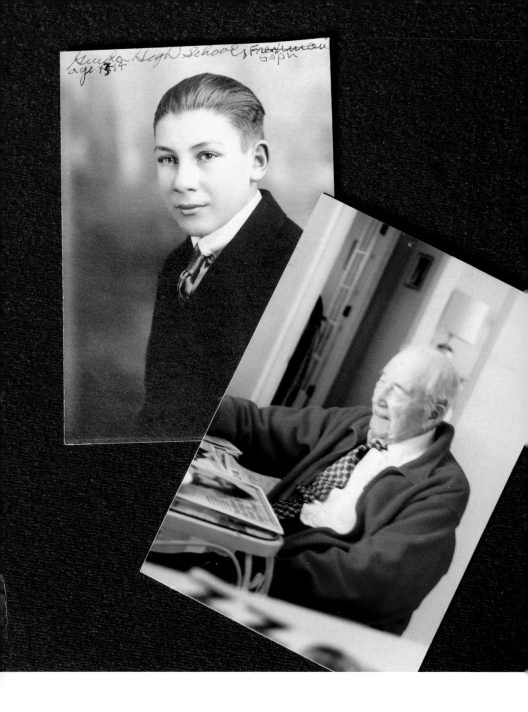

Guido Sartor, the author's father, pictured about the time of the influenza pandemic and, in his 90s, reviewing scenes from this book.